Clinical Protocols

*a guide for nurses
and physicians*

Clinical Protocols

a guide for nurses and physicians

Carolyn M. Hudak, R.N., M.S.
Assistant Professor of Nursing and Medicine
Adult Nurse Practitioner
University of Colorado Medical Center

Paul M. Redstone, M.D.
Assistant Professor of Medicine
University of Colorado Medical Center

Nancy L. Hokanson, R.N., M.N.
Adult Nurse Practitioner
Instructor/Adult Nurse Practitioner Program
School of Nursing
University of Colorado Medical Center

Irene E. Suzuki, R.N., M.S.
Adult Nurse Practitioner
University of Colorado Medical Center

J. B. Lippincott Company
Philadelphia
New York   San Jose   Toronto

Distributed in Great Britain by
Blackwell Scientific Publications
London   Oxford   Edinburgh

ISBN 0-397-54179-1
Library of Congress Catalog Card Number 75-43685

Printed in the United States of America
2   4   6   8   9   7   5   3

Library of Congress Cataloging in Publication Data

Main entry under title:

Clinical protocols: a guide for nurses and physicians.

Includes bibliographies and index.
1. Medical protocols.   2. Medicine, Clinical—
Handbooks, manuals, etc.   I. Hudak, Carolyn M.
[DNLM: 1. Medical history taking.   2. Ambulatory
care WB290 C641]
RC64.C55   616'.026   75-43685
ISBN 0-397-54179-1

Contributing Authors

Ernestine K. Dunn, R.N.
Adult Nurse Practitioner
University of Colorado Medical Center

Kathleen L. Headrick, R.N., B.S.
Adult Nurse Practitioner
University of Colorado Medical Center

Jacqueline M. Heppler, R.N., M.S.
Geriatric Nurse Practitioner
Assistant Professor
School of Nursing
University of Colorado

Anne C. Murray, R.N., M.S.
Adult Nurse Practitioner
University of Colorado Medical Center

Lois M. Raday, R.N., B.S.N.
Associate in Practice with
Harold L. Dobson, M.D.,
Houston, Texas
Formerly Adult Nurse Practitioner
University of Colorado Medical Center

Judith A. Rottink, R.N., B.S.
Adult Nurse Practitioner
University of Colorado Medical Center

E. June Watkins, R.N.
Adult Nurse Practitioner
University of Colorado Medical Center

Special Editor

Sonia M. Flanders, R.N., M.S.N.
Head Nurse Clinician
Medical Outpatient Department
University of Colorado Medical Center

Acknowledgments

We thank the nurses and physicians of the Colorado General Hospital Medical Clinics who supported the development of the adult nurse practitioner role in this area and who recognized the need for protocols of this type.

We also thank Ms. Barbara Haab Fluitt for her superior performance in typing the manuscript from exceptionally rough drafts.

Dedication

To those practitioners who pioneered the role and those who will continue to develop it

Preface

This book evolved from our experience as practitioners and educators in an ambulatory adult care setting within a major medical center. Because the medical and nursing staff in this area are closely involved with nurse practitioner training in association with the University of Colorado Schools of Nursing and Medicine, our clinic settings are a primary clinical practice area for students. The practitioners in this setting recognized a need for guidelines to handle common patient problems, not only for teaching purposes, but as a starting point to guarantee a standardized level of care for patients.

As a result of the University of Colorado's pioneering efforts in developing the nurse practitioner role, we have had frequent requests for patient care protocols to serve as initial guides for others. On the basis of these requests, we decided to develop protocols for the problems most commonly seen in our setting.

The Medical Clinics of the University of Colorado Outpatient Department encompass areas for the continuing care of patients with general medical or medical subspecialty problems and an Adult Walk-In Clinic, a non-appointment clinic for patients with acute, self-limiting problems. The Adult Walk-In Clinic is staffed by six nurse practitioners and a medical resident who see the majority of patients coming to this area. An attending physician is available for consultation.

The acute problem protocols developed for this book are based on the most common presenting complaints seen in this setting, while the chronic disease protocols include those conditions most often followed by the nurse practitioner in a continuing care clinic. We have attempted to define an appropriate data base for the common acute problems as well as the chronic illnesses which nurse practitioners may be managing. The protocol material is presented in a problem-oriented framework, outlining the subjective and objective data, detailing some of the more common conditions causing a given presenting complaint and including diagnostic, therapeutic and patient education aspects of the plan. Since we strongly believe that the nurse practitioner's practice must evolve from a sound knowledge base, the rationale is described for each piece of the data base outlined in the worksheet. The material in the rationale is organized in the same sequence as the worksheet items. This feature should increase the book's usefulness as a resource for the experienced practitioner while serving as an educational guide for the student.

It is important to emphasize that the protocols are intended only to serve as *guides* for other practice settings. Other practitioners will need to test and modify them according to the special characteristics of their setting and patient population. Also, the reader is cautioned not to view the assessment components of the protocols as absolutes. The experienced practitioner is aware that patients do not fit into boxes and to limit one's thinking or categorize patient problems can be hazardous. Instead, we have provided some initial data on common problems and encourage the reader to refer to specialty texts when more specific or inclusive information is needed.

A chapter is devoted to Health Maintenance since this is a key area of nursing practice. The concepts of health and illness are closely interfaced in the adult. Because the majority of health care seeking behavior is still prompted by illness, the nurse practitioner must utilize each patient encounter for education in ways to maintain health and reduce risk for potential illness.

Although the primary focus of this book is the nurse practitioner in practice and the nurse practitioner student, the protocols may also be useful to other health professionals as a starting point for defining levels of care. Use of this book assumes a fundamental knowledge of history taking and physical assessment skills.

The size and format of the book is designed to encourage maximum utilization by the practitioner. Space is provided at the end of each protocol so the practitioner can note additional data as his/her knowledge base expands. It is also designed so that it may be easily carried to serve as a resource when seeing patients.

It is our hope that the ultimate outcome of the book will be the translation of its information into meaningful data for use in patient education by the practitioner.

Carolyn M. Hudak
Paul M. Redstone
Nancy L. Hokanson
Irene E. Suzuki

Contents

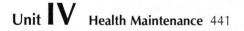

Introduction to protocols for practice

Chapter 1

Development
and utilization
of protocols

The term "protocol" is subject to a variety of interpretations nowadays but for our purposes it is defined as an organized method of analyzing and dealing with a disease process or symptom complex. A protocol may be highly organized and directive, as in some algorithms, or it may be more general and flexible. The type selected for development and use will depend on the clinical practice situation, the education and experience of those who will be using the protocol and the availability of physician support. A minimally trained person who has limited physician availability will require a protocol that is very explicit, whereas a more highly trained professional may require only general guidelines, particularly if physician consultation is available when necessary.

The initial development of protocols is no easy task, as you may already know from your own attempts. When a number of people are involved in the initial work, the task can become fairly complex. However, it is important that those who will be using the protocols have input into their development. Protocols, as we envision them, should reflect mutual effort by the nurse practitioner/physician team. Once developed and in use, a plan must be outlined for their periodic revision by the team. This periodic updating is important for several reasons:

1. Your experience may show that certain important data are missing or that some data being collected are superfluous.
2. New knowledge may become available and should be included.
3. Previous knowledge may be proved incorrect.
4. Experience may demonstrate that an entity dealt with in one pro-

tocol is too broad and actually should be covered in two or more, e.g. URI protocol may need to be separated into:
1. sinusitis
2. otitis media

Because the format of a protocol is determined by its purpose, the purposes behind the protocols in this book deserve some elaboration. Primarily, these protocols are intended to serve as a resource and teaching guide for nurse practitioners. Thus, they are more detailed than one might normally find and include the rationale for each item listed in the data base and plan. Our intent is to provide an increased understanding about the given problems so that the nurse practitioner might have a sound basis to guide and defend her actions, as well as to use in the education of patients.

The protocols assume a background of nursing theory and history-taking and physical assessment skills. For this reason, they require a rather sophisticated level of judgment in their implementation.

Keep in mind that a protocol developed for one setting cannot automatically be transferred to a different setting. Consequently, the protocols presented here must be individualized to the particular setting in which they will be used and to the special characteristics of the health professionals who will use them. Health professionals do not always agree on the criteria and management of a given problem; therefore, these and other protocols will be subject to challenge. For this reason, protocols should be considered experimental and tested for validity in a given practice setting.

Regardless of a protocol's specificity, its use has some distinct advantages over performance that is solely memory based:

A PROTOCOL:

1. *Provides a consistent data base.* Once the nurse practitioner/physician team has agreed upon what is important to ask and do for a particular problem, the protocol helps insure that these data are collected in every appropriate patient encounter. It also helps the practitioner collect the data in a more organized and consistent fashion.
2. *Helps insure thoroughness.* Assuming that the data base outlined in a given protocol is complete, using the protocol during a patient encounter should insure that no significant information is forgotten by the examiner.
3. *Is convenient.* A long checklist may at first seem quite imposing. However, once a practitioner becomes familiar with a protocol, col-

lection of the data base is actually facilitated. This occurs because there is no delay in thinking about what to do or ask next, and usually there is less writing involved.

4. *Facilitates audit of care and performance.* After a consistent data base has been established, it becomes relatively easy to evaluate the thoroughness and reliability of the care-giver. Inconsistencies in performance can be identified, thus providing an educational experience for the practitioner and directly influencing patient care.

5. *Encourages continued learning.* The initial development of a protocol is a great learning experience. The research, conferences and decision-making involved in setting up a protocol are invaluable to all those who participate. And, once developed, opportunities for learning continue during the testing and subsequent revision of the protocol.

The major arguments against the use of protocols contend that they force the practitioners into a predetermined mode of operation, thus stifling clinical judgments, and that protocols do not recognize the uniqueness of individual patients. It is our feeling that if the practitioner is involved in creating and revising the protocol, any apparent limitations can be identified and remedied. It is precisely the uniqueness of each individual that demands high level judgment on the part of the health professional in any patient encounter. The value of any protocol is in many ways dependent upon the person using it. However, we believe that protocols, properly utilized, can lead to better patient care.

Chapter 2

Use of descriptors
and the
general systems review

Throughout the protocols in this book, symptoms elicited in the history are further expanded by use of what we refer to as "descriptors." Many of these descriptors, such as location, radiation and character, were orginally developed for the description of pain. However, these and others can often be applied to all other symptoms. The use of a set of descriptors is helpful in setting up a standard data base. Their use encourages thoroughness, as the practitioner has a consistent framework from which to evaluate many different symptoms. The first part of this chapter will be devoted to explaining the descriptors in some detail so that the reader can become more familiar with their use and apply them in the protocols. An outline, with examples, is given at the end of this section.

The second part of the chapter will consist of a general outline of a complete "Review of Systems." This second part is not meant to be inclusive of all possible symptoms, and it is beyond the scope of this text to elaborate on the possible causes of each of the symptoms. The outline is meant only as a reference and starting point to allow the practitioner to expand his/her inquiry into areas that may not be detailed in the specific protocol. This is particularly important if, in use of one of the protocols, the nurse practitioner finds that the patient's problem may well be in another area. In general, an entire review of systems will not be gone through with each patient seen for the common problems described in the protocols. The entire review of systems is generally done only when a patient is being evaluated with a complete history and physical.

Descriptors

Time relationships. One of the most important and sometimes most difficult things to find out about a patient's complaint is when it actually began. It is important to encourage the patient to recall the initial onset of the symptoms. Associated with this, it is important to determine what the patient was doing at the time the symptoms began. Was the onset abrupt or gradual? What is the duration of the symptoms? What is their frequency of occurrence? How long has each of these recurrences lasted? Have the frequency, duration and mode of onset of the complaint changed at all since it first began? All of these points are important in gaining a clear idea about the nature of the complaint.

Location. This descriptor finds its greatest usefulness in the description of pain. You must insist that the patient give you an accurate location of the pain. A good way to do this is to have the patient point with one finger to the location of his pain or to where it is most severe. It is felt by many clinicians that inability to point out an area of localization is one characteristic of functional illness.

Radiation. Again, use can be made of the patient's finger to point out the course of his pain and where it goes. It must also be remembered that occasionally pain can be present in the area of radiation with little or no pain at the site of the pathologic process initiating that pain. Knowledge of the anatomic pathways involved helps enable the practitioner to use pain radiation to accurately pinpoint the source of the problem.

Character. This is one of the most difficult areas to evaluate, as the patient may not even describe his distress or discomfort as an actual pain. An individual's perception of pain is also colored by his past experience, and you must be certain that the words the patient uses to describe his pain are interpreted correctly by you. Such terms as "burning," "sharp," "dull," "aching," "gnawing," "throbbing," "cramping," "vise-like" or "constricting" may mean entirely different things to different people. It is sometimes helpful in this regard to lead the patient, in that you can attempt to compare the character of the pain to the pain experienced during a familiar circumstance, e.g. achy pain as felt during a toothache, sharp pain as felt with a pin or needle, cramping pain as with diarrhea. If you can get through the language barrier, the character of a patient's pain may be invaluable in helping you pinpoint the etiology. *Character* is also useful in describing other things, e.g. stool, sputum.

Associated Factors. This category encompasses all other alterations and experiences associated with the patient's complaint. For example:

With chest pain, has the patient noted associated diaphoresis, dyspnea, nausea or vomiting? Is the patient's vaginal discharge associated with pruritus or lower abdominal pain? Is the frequency of urination associated with chills and fever? It is again important to question the patient and have him volunteer any associated symptoms, but it is also important to ask about specific symptoms if a certain disease is suspected. For example: If you suspect any type of infection, questions about chills, fever and sweats should be asked. Most of the common "associated symptoms" are included on the various protocols. If further investigation is indicated, the appropriate review of systems should be used (see below).

Exacerbating Factors. The patient should be questioned closely about factors which will initiate or worsen his complaints. Is the pain made worse by activity, coughing, breathing? The classic pain of angina pectoris is often said to be initiated by the three E's—eating, emotion and exercise.

Course. It is necessary to determine whether the patient's illness is constant, intermittent, progressing or subsiding. An illness with a progressive course, especially if rapid, requires a more rapid evaluation. Following the course of an illness, e.g. systemic lupus, rheumatoid arthritis, may be the only way a definitive diagnosis can be established.

Alleviating Factors. Closely coupled to those things that exacerbate the patient's problem are those that will relieve it. Is the patient's problem relieved by rest, by sitting or lying in a certain position, by eating certain foods? It is essential that all these factors be recorded even if they don't seem to make particular sense to you at the time of the history. The clues may all fit together in the end.

Effects of Medication. Finally, it is important to question the patient closely as to what medicines he has taken and their effect on his problem. It is imperative to question the patient closely particularly as regards the use of over-the-counter medications such as laxatives or cold remedies. The patient will often not think of these things as actual medicines, and unless questioned specifically about what he has done to try to get relief, he may not even mention them. It is also important to determine those medicines used chronically by the patient, as one of these may be the etiologic agent in his present problem.

Ideally, each of the patient's complaints should be evaluated in the above manner. Often, because of the time constraints imposed upon the practitioner, it is not possible to do this. The patient's chief complaint or complaints should certainly be evaluated in the above manner, and the protocols have generally been designed with this in mind.

In addition, if questioning and examination of the patient reveals the need for further investigation, the patient should be scheduled to return for that purpose.

Outline of Descriptors

TIME RELATIONSHIPS

COMMENCED:

Recently: hours, days, weeks
Long term: 1 month ago, 6 months ago, 1 year ago

ONSET:

Sudden or gradual

NUMBER OF EPISODES:

Intermittent; increasing or decreasing frequency
Occasional

OTHER:

going to sleep	afternoon
meal time	evenings
early a.m.	nocturnal
daytime only	awakens patient

LOCATION–RADIATION

anterior chest	⟶	left arm
right upper quadrant	⟶	right scapula
flank	⟶	groin

CHARACTER

sharp	deep	pressure-like
dull	superficial	crushing
burning		squeezing

Severity at worst:
Marked—completely incapacitated
Moderate—interferes with work
Mild—doesn't interfere with activities

ASSOCIATED WITH

Known diagnosis
Physiological problems
Others, e.g.
diaphoresis, nausea, vomiting, chest pain

PRECIPITATED BY

social circumstances	medicine
position or position change	foods, alcohol
environmental changes	exertion

COURSE

Rapid or slow progression—stable—getting better/worse—not completely subsided—intermittent—fluctuating

RELIEVED BY–NOT RELIEVED BY

position	medication	nothing
sleep	food	
rest	exertion	

Outline of a "Review of Systems"

Following is a list of specific symptoms about which the patient should be questioned when a given body system is evaluated

HEAD: Headache, dizziness, trauma

EYES: Blurred vision, diplopia, lacrimation, burning, dryness, photophobia, scotomata

EARS: Decreased hearing, tinnitus, pain, pruritus, discharge, previous infections

NOSE (including sinuses): Abnormal or absent sense of smell, frequent colds, discharge, obstruction, epistaxis, history of sinusitis, trauma

MOUTH AND THROAT: Bleeding gums, frequent sore throats, sore tongue, poor dentition (caries, abscesses, dentures), dryness, abnormal taste, dysphagia, hoarseness

RESPIRATORY: Cough, sputum, dyspnea, hemoptysis, pleurisy or other chest pain; history of pneumonia, tuberculosis, or asthma; cyanosis, wheezing; date and result of last chest x-ray

CARDIOVASCULAR: Precordial pain or distress, dyspnea, edema, orthopnea, paroxysmal nocturnal dyspnea; history of heart disease, murmur or high blood pressure; claudication, palpitations; nocturia

GASTROINTESTINAL: Abdominal pain or distress, nausea, vomiting, diarrhea, constipation, hematochezia, melena, jaundice, bloating, flatulence, eructation; history of peptic disease, gallbladder disease, inflammatory bowel disease; hemorrhoids; hernia; change in appetite, food intolerance

GENITOURINARY: Frequency, urgency, dysuria, pyuria, polyuria, oliguria, nocturia; renal or ureteral stone and/or colic; testicular pain; hematuria; poor stream, dribbling; history of urinary tract infection

GYNECOLOGICAL: Menarche, menses (frequency, duration, amount of flow), dysmenorrhea, spotting, parity (history of toxemia), date of last menstrual period; breast tenderness or soreness; vaginal discharge

VENEREAL: Urethral or vaginal discharge, sore, ulcer; history of prior disease; gonorrhea (whites, strain, clap); syphilis (bad blood, hair cut, needle treatments)

NEUROMUSCULAR: Seizure, loss of consciousness, anesthesia, paresthesia, neuralgia, twitch, tremor; personality change, memory deficit, mental deterioration; nervousness, anxiety, history of psychiatric problems; muscle weakness, stiffness, soreness; poor coordination or balance

SKELETAL: Arthralgia, arthritis, stiffness, back pain, neck pain, sciatica; heat, swelling, tenderness in any joint

GLANDS: Lymphadenopathy; enlargement or tenderness of thyroid, parotid, lacrimal gland; breast tenderness, enlargement, nipple discharge

ENDOCRINE: Rate of growth, weight change; heat or cold intolerance; abnormal pigmentation, change in skin texture; sweating, flushing, irregular menses; weakness; polydipsia, polyphagia, polyuria

HEMATOLOGICAL: Weakness, pallor, easy bruising, prolonged bleeding, history of anemia

SKIN: Rashes, pruritus, photosensitivity; growths or lumps; change in hair texture or distribution

12

Protocols for common acute self-limiting problems

Introduction to Common Acute Self-Limiting Problem Protocols

The acute problem protocols in this section are based on the most common presenting complaints seen in a general adult ambulatory clinic setting. The protocol material is presented in a problem-oriented framework and outlines the subjective and objective data base in worksheet form. The rationale is then described for each item in the data base and is organized in the same sequence as the worksheet.

The assessment component of these protocols details some of the more common conditions causing a given presenting complaint. No attempt was made to be all-inclusive as the practitioner is encouraged to refer to specialty texts when more specific information is needed. The user is also cautioned not to view the assessment components as absolutes. The uniqueness of each individual must be considered in the application of this information.

The *Subjective and Objective Data* components of the worksheets are set up so that a "Yes" response indicates an abnormality. This format allows the practitioner to quickly identify or review positive findings. Studies included under *Lab Data* are those which are usually quickly obtained and useful in making the assessment of the problem. The *diagnostic* component of the *Plan* includes those studies not immediately available, but which are necessary for further definition of the problem.

The *therapeutic* component of the *Plan* is, in most instances, stated in general categories rather than suggesting specific drugs or dosages. This increases the flexibility of the protocols and allows individual practice settings to define their own specific treatment regimens.

The *patient education* section of the *Plan* is very important, but also very difficult to outline. Some general areas of education are mentioned, but the practitioner will need to expand this section based on the special needs of each patient. The information contained in the *Rationale* can be translated into meaningful patient information for this purpose.

Since the primary purpose of these protocols is to serve as a resource and teaching guide, they are more detailed than the usual protocol. However, as the practitioner gains experience with a particular problem, collection of the data base should become increasingly efficient. Space has been provided at the end of each acute problem protocol so that additional notes can be made.

be considered that which occurs suddenly and without previous recurrent attacks.

Chronic nausea and vomiting is recurrent or continuous over an extended period of time.

BIBLIOGRAPHY

Harvey, A. M., et al.: *The Principles and Practice of Medicine*, 18th ed., New York: Appleton-Century-Crofts, 1972.

MacBryde, C. M. (ed.): *Signs and Symptoms*, 5th ed., Philadelphia: Lippincott, 1970.

Wintrobe, M. W., et al. (eds.): *Harrison's Principles of Internal Medicine*, 7th ed., New York: McGraw Hill, 1974.

NOTES

NOTES

Chapter 4

Abdominal pain

ABDOMINAL PAIN WORKSHEET

To be used in patients with:
Indigestion
Heartburn
Abdominal Pain
Cramps

What you can't afford to miss: "acute abdomen" (origin of pain is perforation, rupture, obstruction, ischemia, generalized inflammation).

Chief Complaint: _____

SUBJECTIVE DATA:

Location of pain (describe): _____

Radiation: _____Yes _____No   If yes, describe: _____

Character of pain, describe: _____

Onset: _____Sudden _____Gradual _____Date of onset

Course: _____Constant _____Progressive

_____Intermittent _____Subsiding

Duration of each episode: _____ Duration of illness:_____

Frequency (number of episodes): _____

Severity at worst: _____

Precipitated by: _____

Made worse by: _____

Relieved by:_____

DESCRIBE POSITIVE RESPONSES
(Include Onset, Severity, Duration)

Yes   *No*

____ ____ Related to activity: _____

____ ____ Related to position:_____

____ ____ Related to meals:_____

____ ____ Related to defecation:_____

____ ____ Related to stress: _____

____ ____ Related to time of day or season: _____

____ ____ Use of aspirin, tea, coffee, alcohol, cigarettes, colas,

bouillon: Circle and describe use: _____

_____

____ ____ Exposure to toxins (specify):

____Foods ____Metals ____Chemicals

____ ____ Unusual water source: _____

ASSOCIATED WITH:
Yes *No*

____ ____ Anorexia: _____

____ ____ Nausea and/or vomiting: _____

____ ____ Change in bowel habits: _____

____ ____ Diarrhea (consistency and color): _____

____ ____ Constipation:_____

____ ____ Blood in stools: _____ Mucus in stools:_____

____ ____ Weight change:_____

____ ____ Flatulence/eructation:_____

____ ____ Bloating:_____

____ ____ Regurgitation/burning: _____

____ ____ Recent trauma: _____

____ ____ Fever/chills: _____

____ ____ Urinary tract symptoms:

_____Dysuria _____

_____Hematuria _____

_____Frequency _____

_____Urgency _____

_____Back pain _____

_____Nocturia _____

_____Other _____

___ ___ Gynecologic symptoms (female only):

     _____Vaginal discharge_____

     _____Genital lesions _____

     _____Irregular bleeding _____

     _____Other _____

     _____Date of last menses

     _____Use of contraceptive:

          _____Intrauterine device

          _____Birth control pill

          _____Other _____

___ ___ Genitourinary symptoms (male only):

     _____Discharge _____

     _____Hernia_____

     _____Scrotal edema, pain_____

     _____Other _____

___ ___ Cardiovascular symptoms (do cardiovascular system

review, if indicated): _____

_____

___ ___ Respiratory symptoms (do respiratory system review, if

indicated): _____

_____

Protocols for Common Acute Self-Limiting Problems

PAST MEDICAL HISTORY:
Yes   No

____ ____ Allergies (describe reaction and source): _____

_____

____ ____ Past history of abdominal pain and/or other gastrointestinal

disease: _____

_____

____ ____ History of serious or chronic illness:_____

_____

____ ____ Family history of gastrointestinal disease (gallbladder,

ulcer, pancreas, liver, cancer): _____

_____

____ ____ Medications: _____

_____

OBJECTIVE DATA:

Vital signs: _____B/P   _____P   _____R   _____T   _____WT

General appearance: _____

Color of skin: _____ Posture:_____

Indication of anxiety, nervousness, depression: _____

_____

DESCRIBE POSITIVE RESPONSES

ABDOMINAL EXAM: ____Not Done

Yes   No

____ ____ Striae, scars, nodules: _____

____ ____ Asymmetry: _____

____ ____ Engorged veins: _____

____ ____ Arterial pulsations: _____

____ ____ Ecchymosis: _____

____ ____ Bowel sounds increased, decreased or absent: _____

_____

____ ____ Bruits (location): _____

____ ____ Friction rubs: _____

____ ____ Liver palpable: _____

____ ____ Spleen palpable: _____

____ ____ Masses: _____

____ ____ Bulging flanks, shifting dullness, fluid wave: _____

_____

____ ____ Tenderness: _____

____ ____ Rebound tenderness (describe): _____

_____

____ ____ Rigidity or guarding (describe): _____

_____

___ ___ Iliopsoas test positive: _____

___ ___ Costovertebral angle tenderness: _____

___ ___ Spine tenderness, spasms, decreased range of motion:

_____

___ ___ Inguinal nodes palpated:

___Enlarged ___Tender ___Red

RECTAL EXAM: ___Not Done
Yes   *No*

___ ___ External hemorrhoids: _____

___ ___ Fistula, abscess: _____

___ ___ Abnormal sphincter tone: _____

___ ___ Tenderness: _____

___ ___ Prostatic tenderness: _____

___ ___ Mass: _____

___ ___ Stool obtained: ___Color ___Hematest

PELVIC EXAM: ___Not Done
Yes   *No*

___ ___ Urethra swollen/inflamed:_____

___ ___ Vulvar lesions: _____

___ ___ Vaginal discharge: ___Color ___Amount

___ ___ Vaginal lesions: _____

___ ___ Cervical erosion/lesions: _____

___ ___ Cervical tenderness: _____

___ ___ Adnexal tenderness/enlargement: _____

___ ___ Masses/fullness: _____

___ ___ Bladder palpable: _____

___ ___ Suprapubic tenderness: _____

___ ___ Other: _____

GENITOURINARY EXAM: ____Not Done
Yes *No*

___ ___ Urethral discharge: _____Color _____Amount

___ ___ External genitalia lesions:_____

___ ___ Scrotal enlargement/tenderness: _____

___ ___ Hernia: _____

___ ___ Bladder palpable: _____

___ ___ Suprapubic tenderness: _____

CARDIOVASCULAR EXAM: ____Not Done
Yes *No*

___ ___ Precordial pulsations: _____ PMI:_____

___ ___ Murmur:_____

___ ___ Extra sounds: _____

___ ___ Arrhythmias: _____

___ ___ Edema: _____

___ ___ Peripheral pulses abnormal:_____

Protocols for Common Acute Self-Limiting Problems

CHEST EXAM: ____Not Done
Yes   No

____ ____ Respiratory restrictions: _____

____ ____ Decreased diaphragm movement: _____

____ ____ Dullness: _____

____ ____ Fremitus increased/decreased: _____

____ ____ Tenderness: _____

____ ____ Rales, rhonchi, wheezes: _____

LAB DATA:
Done Not
*   Done*

____ ____ CBC: ____HGB ____HCT ____WBC ____ESR

____ ____ Urinalysis: ____pH ____Bilirubin ____Protein

                    ____Glucose ____Ketones ____Blood

                    ____Bacteria ____RBC ____WBC

                    ____Casts ____Crystals ____Gravindex

____ ____ Vaginal or urethral discharge:

                    _____Wet prep _____Gram stain

____ ____ Enzymes: _____Amylase _____Lipase

____ ____ Liver function: _____SGOT _____SGPT

____ ____ X-Rays: _____Chest

                    _____Abdominal

                    _____Other

___ ___ Electrocardiogram: _____

___ ___ Other: _____

ASSESSMENT:

_____

_____

_____

_____

PLAN:

_____ Consultation: _____

_____ Admit to hospital

DIAGNOSTIC:

_____ X-Rays

_____ Oral cholecystogram

_____ Upper gastrointestinal exam

_____ Barium enema

_____ Intravenous pyelogram

_____ Sigmoidoscopy

_____ Other: _____

Protocols for Common Acute Self-Limiting Problems

_____Culture

    _____Urine

    _____Cervical for gonorrhea

    _____Stool:

        _____Bacteria

        _____Ova and parasites

_____Bloods

    _____Lipase

    _____Liver function tests

    _____Australia antigen

    _____Other: _____

THERAPEUTIC:

    _____Antiemetic: _____

    _____Analgesic: _____

    _____Laxative:_____

    _____Antidiarrheic: _____

    _____Antacid: _____

    _____Anticholinergic: _____

    _____Tranquilizer:_____

    _____Diet: _____

    _____Other: _____

PATIENT EDUCATION:

_____Medications: _____

_____Diet: _____

_____Rest:_____

_____Decrease use of gastric irritants:_____

_____Reduce risk factors:_____

_____Identify situational stress:_____

_____Refer to other clinic: _____

_____Call for test results:_____

_____Return to clinic: _____

_____Other: _____

ABDOMINAL PAIN

There are many conditions arising from both the intra-abdominal cavity and extra-abdominal areas which can first present as abdominal pain. "Acute abdomen" is an all-encompassing term defined as any abdominal disease process which requires immediate treatment, whether surgical or medical. It is the "acute abdomen" which one cannot afford to miss in evaluating a patient with abdominal pain. Examples of acute abdomen involving the GI tract include perforated ulcer, appendicitis and complete bowel obstruction. Additionally, life-threatening situations arising from other body systems can first present as abdominal pain. Among these are myocardial infarction, dissecting aortic aneurysm and ruptured ectopic pregnancy.

In general, the situation is of immediate concern if the origin of the abdominal pain is perforation, rupture, obstruction, ischemia, generalized peritonitis or a condition that may in the immediate future lead to one of these conditions.

Abdominal pain can also be the presenting complaint for persons with chronic or long-term conditions as well as with emotional or psychiatric problems. These conditions, although not immediately life threatening, could lead to more serious problems and they deserve thorough investigation.

The etiology of abdominal pain can be summarized as:[1]

ORIGINATING WITHIN THE ABDOMEN

1. Diseases of hollow organs: bowel, gallbladder, ducts, etc.

2. Peritonitis: chemical or bacterial

3. Vascular: mesenteric thrombosis, dissecting aneurysm, etc.

4. Tension on supporting structures or distention of capsules (spleen, liver, lymph nodes, etc.)

ORIGINATING OUTSIDE THE ABDOMEN

1. Referred pain from thorax, spine, spinal cord, pelvis, genitourinary tract, etc.

2. Metabolic pain
   a. Endogenous such as allergic reactions, uremia, diabetic acidosis, food hypersensitivity, sickle cell disease, porphyria
   b. Exogenous; chemicals and toxic drugs, bacterial toxins

3. Neurogenic pain

4. Psychogenic pain

ABDOMINAL PAIN WORKSHEET RATIONALE

SUBJECTIVE DATA:

Location of pain, with and without Radiation

Unfortunately, abdominal pain described by the patient as being in one specific area does not *always* coincide with organs found in that region of the abdomen. However, a good starting point in evaluating the origin of the pain is to keep in

[1]MacBryde, C. M. (ed.): *Signs and Symptoms,* 5th ed., Philadelphia: Lippincott, 1970, p. 187.

mind organs which are in the general area of the pain described.

Epigastric pain	Origin may be duodenal or gastric, gallbladder, pancreas, high small bowel or gastric outlet, renal, liver, thoracic, cardiac, appendix or mesenteric arterial ischemia.
Epigastric-midsternal pain with or without radiation to neck/shoulders	Origin may be hiatal hernia with esophageal reflux or myocardial infarction.
Periumbilical or mid-abdominal pain	Origin may be appendix, small bowel, pancreas or stomach.
Lower abdominal and suprapubic pain	Origin may be colon, appendix, adnexal, bladder or uterus.
Epigastric pain radiating to back or shoulders	May be associated with pancreatic, peptic ulcer, hiatal hernia, subphrenic abscess or diaphragmatic origin. Myocardial infarction pain may present this way or may also radiate to one or both arms.
Right upper quadrant pain radiating to midscapular area of back	Associated with gallbladder disease.
Upper quadrant or costovertebral angle pain radiating to acromial, lower cervical area or more commonly to inguinal or genital area	Associated with kidney or ureter disease.
Left upper quadrant pain	Origin may be spleen or splenic flexure of colon.
Epigastric pain migrating to right lower quadrant	Associated with the appendix.

Pain Character

The quality of the pain can help determine what process or mechanism for pain is involved as well as help determine what organ or structure is involved. Mechanisms for pain produced in the abdomen include:

1. Distention of tubes, vessels and viscera.
2. Vigorous contraction of smooth muscle.
3. Inflammation of the peritoneum.
4. Peritoneal stretching.
5. Distention of the vascular system.
6. Ischemia.
7. Spinal root and peripheral nerve irritation or inflammation.
8. Sustained contraction of skeletal muscle or other processes in the abdominal wall.
9. Unknown processes.

Constant pain

Usually caused by inflammation, marked swelling or overdistention of solid viscus such as liver, spleen or kidney.

Localized pain

Pain is usually of parietal peritoneum origin where pain fibers are close to the skin and thus more easily localized by the patient.

Dull ache or generalized burning

Indicates deep visceral or deep somatic structure involvement. These structures have fewer pain fibers and are innervated by fibers from both sides of the spinal cord. Thus, the pain is more diffuse.

Colicky with pain-free intervals

Caused by mechanical obstruction of the stomach, intestine or colon.

The more proximal the obstruction the shorter the pain-free interval; the more distal the obstruction the longer the pain-free interval.

Colicky pain without free intervals

May subside cyclically but is never absent. This occurs late in obstruction of a hollow viscus as with biliary or renal stones, high small bowel obstruction and intestinal strangulation. Major peaks correlate with increased muscular activity of the obstructed viscus; lesser peaks are due to ischemia.

Cramps

Indicates involvement of a hollow viscus with early inflammation, irritation or obstruction. When more serious intra-abdominal disease occurs, cramps may change to colic or to a constant ache.

Migratory pain

Is due to involvement of different tissues at various stages of the disease process.

Referred pain which is sharp and localized

This is a viscerosensory reflex secondary to neurons excited in the cord so communication is opened between afferent visceral fibers and somatic dermatomes. Usually means inflammation of an organ and/or added inflammation of parietal peritoneum or mesentery. Referred pain can also follow embryologic pathways of organs.

Onset and Course of Pain

Generally, sudden onset of pain requires immediate evaluation, whereas gradual onset indicates a chronic process. However, this is not always true, and one particularly needs to be aware of changes in the course of the pain. Pain that progressively worsens would indicate extended involvement of the disease process.

Severity at Worst

It is difficult for patients to describe pain and its severity. It may be helpful to relate the severity to something known, such as smashing a finger, having teeth pulled, etc. One can also rate the pain on a scale of 1-10, 10 being the most severe. How the pain interferes with the patient's activities of daily living can also help determine severity.

Precipitated by, Relieved by, Made Worse by

Related to activity and position

Pain may be exacerbated or precipitated by movement in the following conditions: perforated ulcer, extrapelvic appendicitis, diverticulitis, renal calculus, biliary colic or peritonitis. Pain of myocardial ischemia is precipitated by exercise, whereas esophageal pain is not. However, esophageal reflux pain may be worsened by bending over or lying flat.

Related to meals

The classic history of acute peptic ulcer pain includes the pain-eat-relief series of events. Also, any food may precipitate the pain in a given individual because of individual food intolerances. Gastric ulcer pain usually begins 30-90 minutes after a meal and duodenal pain begins 2-4 hours after a meal. This pain often persists until the next meal. Large meals with roughage may precipitate the pain of diverticulitis, while enteritis pain may be precipitated by anything eaten. Large meals may cause distention and thus stimulate the release of gastrin which in turn stimulates the release of acid. Pain of mesenteric vascular insufficiency gets worse 15 minutes to 3 hours after eating, and is in proportion to the size of the meal. Chronic peptic ulcer disease can present differently than acute peptic ulcer disease. Eating can aggravate pain, as scarring of the mucosa in the duodenum may block emptying of food from the stomach.

Related to defecation

Pain of ulcerative colitis and regional enteritis may be relieved by defecation.

Related to stress

One needs to be aware of stress in relation to work or family situations. Stress can be the cause of pain but can also precipitate pain with an organic basis. Irritable colon represents about 50 % of all gastrointestinal illnesses; it is an example of bodily adaptation to nonspecific stress. Ulcerative colitis and regional enteritis have a relationship to stress, as does peptic ulcer disease.

Time of day or season

One way to differentiate between organic pain and functional pain is to determine whether the pain disappears at night and sleep is undisturbed. Organic pain does not know the time of day. Other considerations include a relationship to seasons due to allergies, and activities at certain times of the day or week related to emotional stress. Peptic ulcer disease in some people becomes worse in the spring and fall but the etiology of this phenomenon is unknown.

Use of gastrointestinal irritants

Gastrointestinal irritants which increase gastric secretions include broth, smoking, alcohol and caffeine-containing drinks such as coffee, tea and colas. Aspirin directly irritates the gastric mucosa.

Exposure to toxins

Chemicals: Exposure to paint, cleaning fluids or insecticides may have a relationship to the pain. Lead and mercury are absorbed by the alimentary tract, and lead ingestion may result in intermittent, vague discomfort, while mercuric chloride causes epigastric pain within minutes after ingestion.

Water source

Contaminated water may be the source of protozoan or bacterial infection.

Associated with
Anorexia

A patient with good appetite is unlikely to have serious gastrointestinal disease.

Nausea and/or vomiting

Caused by the activation of the emetic center in the medulla oblongata by way of afferent impulses arising in the GI tract. Impulses are principally those in the vagus and splanchnic nerves. Hematemesis indicates GI tract bleeding. Bright red blood means recent hemorrhage, and coffee ground appearance occurs when the digestive processes change the hemoglobin to brown pigment; this may take only a few minutes. Time relationship of nausea and vomiting to the pain is also important:

Peptic ulcer: nausea and vomiting is very common and may relieve the pain.

Pyloric obstruction: vomiting of undigested food occurs up to 12 hours after meals.

Ulcer perforation and peritonitis: the vomiting and retching that occurs with an ulcer may stop but recurs with perforation and peritonitis.

Obstruction of small bowel: vomiting is most prominent with a high obstruction; may become feculent with lower obstruction.

Obstruction of large bowel: nausea is present but vomiting may not be.

Appendicitis: nausea and vomiting may be present but not persistent.

Pancreatitis: there is incessant retching, often bilious.

Cholecystitis: vomiting is slight unless stone enters the duct or peritonitis develops.

Change in bowel habits: diarrhea or constipation blood in stools

Any change in bowel habits is significant and history of such change needs to be explored. Examples of causes for bowel changes are as follows:

Melena: present with bleeding proximal to the ligament of Treitz.

Bright red rectal bleeding: indicates lower gastrointestinal tract hemorrhage or massive upper GI tract hemorrhage.

Constipation: present with bowel obstruction, which may be incomplete, and with cholecystitis. A long history of constipation with intervals of diarrhea may indicate diverticulosis, functional bowel syndrome, or bowel tumor. A recent change in bowel habits, particularly an increase in constipation, occurs with cancer of the rectum, sigmoid and descending colon. Rectal bleeding usually occurs with rectal lesions such as cancer.

Diarrhea: may precede appendicitis, but is not usually present during attack. Chronic diarrhea is present with regional enteritis as well as with ulcerative colitis. Diarrhea is frequently nocturnal with colitis. Diarrhea may also occur with distal colonic lesions such as tumor or impaction.

Weight change

Any change of weight is noteworthy if patient is not dieting. Early satiety may indicate carcinoma of the stomach. Loss of weight could be indicator of processes such as malabsorption, cancer or colitis.

Flatulence/eructation/ bloating

This indicates an increase in gas in the GI tract. The patient could be an air swallower, the air causing distention of the viscera. Bacteria and other organisms such as Giardia can also produce increased gas. Flatulence along with bloating is often seen with enteritis and is common with appendicitis and diverticulitis. Patients may complain of "gas" or a full feeling with cancer of the stomach, and persons with angina pectoris may attribute pain to "gas."

Regurgitation/heartburn

A midsternal burning sensation is the most common clinical manifestation of esophageal reflux. Regurgitation occurs later with esophageal reflux when gastric contents pass the gastroesophageal sphincter and escape into the esophagus in the absence of belching or vomiting.

Recent trauma

This could be the cause of internal injury such as ruptured spleen.

Fever/chills

Usually indicates an infectious process.

Urinary tract symptoms

These symptoms point to urinary tract origin of the pain such as infection or calculus. See Dysuria Protocol.

Gynecological symptoms

History of vaginal bleeding and/or discharge may point to acute salpingitis, vaginitis or venereal disease. Tubal pregnancy also needs to be ruled out.

Genitourinary symptoms

Urethritis or venereal disease may be the cause of pain. Testicular pain is present with epididymitis. Infection of the seminal vesicle may cause radiation of pain into the pelvis. Hernia may lead to bowel strangulation.

Cardiovascular symptoms

Angina pectoris or myocardial infarction pain may be referred to sternal or epigastric region. The patient may attribute the pain to gaseous distention. In heart failure the increased extraction of oxygen from blood in the splanchnic area can cause an anoxic state in the liver. This leads to edema and fatty changes in the liver lobule and atrophy and necrosis of hepatic cells surrounding central veins, which leads to pooled blood and hepatomegaly. Stretching of the liver capsule causes right upper quadrant pain which is a constant ache or colic. This is a common sign of congestive heart failure.

The arteries supplying blood to the abdominal viscera branch off the aorta. Thus, with dissecting aneurysm of the aorta, pain can mimic an acute abdominal crisis. The pain may shift to a lower body level as the dissection extends.

Respiratory symptoms

When the diaphragmatic surfaces of the pleura are inflamed, pain may be referred to the abdomen. This occurs when the intercostal innervation of the diaphragm is involved during pneumonia.

With pulmonary embolism or infarction or cancer of the lung, the patient may have abdominal pain along the costal margin. Pleurisy can also present as abdominal pain.

Past Medical History

Allergies

This may alter the plan of care as well as indicate the origin of pain if having allergic reaction to drugs, foods, pollen, etc.

Past gastrointestinal history

History of abdominal surgery, gastrointestinal illness, x-ray exams and treatment are important as they may eliminate or increase suspicion for current specific problems. Examples are: gallbladder and peptic disease, cancer, diverticula, colitis.

History of serious or chronic illness

History of other illnesses, even though not gastrointestinal, may give clues to the patient's underlying disorder.

Family history

History of familial gastrointestinal problems may give clues to the patient's disorder. Specifics to look for are: gallbladder disease, ulcers, pancreatic problems, liver problems and cancer.

Medications

It is important to identify these as they may play an etiological or complicating role in the patient's illness.

OBJECTIVE DATA:

Vital signs

Can detect infectious process or signs of shock (postural changes in blood pressure) with hemorrhage or perforation. With dissecting aneurysm, lower extremity pulses may be decreased or absent.

The pulse will usually be normal in early acute abdominal pain; a progressive increase may indicate intra-abdominal infection or perforation. In the early stages of a "surgical abdomen" the temperature usually stays normal. A slight increase (99-100° F.) may be present with appendicitis. A patient with acute pancreatitis will usually have only a slight fever. When the temperature gets as high as 103-104° F., fluctuates and is accompanied with chills, it is indicative of abscess or rupture. A patient with salpingitis will often have a fever of 103-104° F.; urinary tract infections or pulmonary infections are also accompanied with temperatures in the range of 104° F.

General appearance/ posture/color of skin

A patient with colic pain may be writhing, twisting and doubled up. A patient with peritonitis will be lying supine and still. Jaundice may be present with liver involvement.

Anxiety/nervousness/ depression

Indicator of general emotional status.

Weight

Weight loss occurs with carcinoma of the bowel and stomach and with colitis and malabsorption states. Weight loss is accompanied by generalized weakness. Hiatal hernia is often present in overweight people.

Abdominal Exam
Inspection
Striae

These are due to prolonged stretching of the skin which causes rupture of the elastic fibers in the reticular layer of the cutis. They may result from tumor, ascites, pregnancy, edema or obesity.

Scars	If present, one needs to elicit information about past trauma or surgery.
Nodules/lesions/bulges	May be first evidence of widespread hematogenous metastases of an internal malignancy.
	Lesions of herpes zoster follow unilateral dermatomes.
	Bulges may indicate presence of hernias.
Asymmetry	Symmetrical enlargement is found in pregnancy, large cysts, ascites, obesity or gaseous distention. An asymmetrical enlargement may be due to obstruction of the bowel, tumor or spinal curvature. Alteration of the normal curves of the back may be caused by infection of the perirenal tissue or a kidney tumor.
Engorged veins	Indicative of obstruction of the inferior vena cava or the portal vein.
Arterial pulsations	May be transmitted to the surface by a solid mass overlying the aorta. They are normally seen in a thin abdomen.
Ecchymosis	May be present with ruptured abdominal aneurysm or any retroperitoneal bleeding.
Auscultation Bowel sounds	Decreased or absent peristaltic sounds indicate motility of the bowel is inhibited by inflammation, gangrene or reflex ileus.

Sounds increased in intensity and frequency may be caused by increased intestinal motility due to diarrhea, laxatives, gastroenteritis and possibly bleeding peptic ulcer. Sounds increased in intensity and frequency may be caused also by intestinal contents being squeezed through a stenotic area. With small intestinal obstruction, there are peristaltic rushes heard simultaneously with abdominal cramping. With mucosal irritation, the increased sounds are not heard in rushes and are of lesser intensity.

Arterial bruits

The presence of a murmur in an abdominal vessel is caused by turbulent flow in a dilated, tortuous or constricted artery. May be heard over an aortic aneurysm.

Venous hums

Although often heard normally in the adult, can also be heard continuously about the umbilicus in the presence of obstructed portal circulation.

Peritoneal friction rubs

May indicate peritoneal lesions. The spleen and the liver are the most common sites for these friction rubs as in splenic infarction or hepatic tumor or abscess.

Percussion

Normal percussion sounds of the abdomen may vary in the presence of:
1. Enlarged organs or atrophic organs, the area of dullness being either increased or decreased.
2. Masses which cause increased areas of dullness.

Spine tenderness, spasms, decreased mobility

Spinal column and spinal cord problems can be referred as abdominal pain; e.g. osteoarthritis of the spine.

Inguinal nodes

If enlarged and/or tender, they may be indicators of an infectious process in the pelvis or legs.

Rectal Exam

Cancer of the bowel is a high ranking cause of death. About 40 % of cancer of the large bowel occurs within reach of the finger with a rectal exam, and one can detect an indurated disc or a protuberant ulcerated growth. Fissures and rectal abscesses can also be detected with a rectal exam. Rectal tenderness may be present in diverticulitis and regional enteritis. With ulcerative colitis the rectum may be spastic and the exam quite uncomfortable. The prostate may be tender or enlarged in the presence of prostatitis. With tenesmus the sphincter tone may be spastic. The stool should be examined for blood and mucus, consistency and color.

Pelvic Exam

This is indicated to rule out gynecological origin of the pain. Localized pelvic tenderness and cervical discharge may indicate salpingitis or endometritis. Pelvic infections, including gonorrhea, may cause abdominal pain.

Genitourinary Exam

Infection of the seminal vesicle may cause pain to radiate to the pelvis; an edematous and tender testicle may indicate epididymitis. Discharge may indicate an infectious process such as gonorrhea.

3. Free fluid in the abdominal ca
ity which causes dullness
flanks that shifts with positio

4. Free air or increased air in
gut which gives tympany.

Palpation

In general, with palpation one
1. Detect and evaluate spasms
tender areas of the abdom
wall.
2. Examine organs—their posi
size, consistency and mobil
3. Detect abnormal masses or f

Tenderness

Spasticity and tenderness
McBurney's point is indicati
appendicitis. With pain of ab
nal origin, pressure on the op
side may increase the pain, w
in thoracically referred pai
pressure will not be painf
bound tenderness is preser
inflammation or irritation
peritoneum.

Rigidity

Peritonitis presents with
like" rigidity. Involuntary
rigidity indicates peritone
tion either infectious or ne

Iliopsoas test

Extension of the leg pre
pain due to irritation of tl
iliopsoas muscle cause
flamed or perforated extra
pendix.

Costovertebral
tenderness

Tenderness over the kidr
to urinary tract infection
caused by an inflamed
overlying the ureters.

Cause of the pain could be a hernia. The origin of pain may be the urinary tract; for example, infection of the urethra, bladder or kidneys.

Cardiovascular Exam

See subjective information for rationale. Also see Chest Pain Protocol.

Congestive heart failure

Congestive heart failure may cause hepatic congestion, hepatomegaly and abdominal pain secondary to stretching of the liver capsule. With dissecting aneurysm the blood pressure may be elevated because of the pre-existing hypertension, but the patient may have the appearance of being in shock. Peripheral arterial occlusion occurs within hours of the dissection. There may be murmurs, weakness of the lower extremeties caused by ischemia or a precordial thrust from left ventricular hypertrophy due to pre-existing hypertension.

Chest Exam

With pulmonary disease such as pneumonia, there will be signs of consolidation, effusion, etc. With diaphragmatic pleurisy, there may be rectus muscle spasm as well. Increased respiratory rate, localized pulmonary signs and absence of rebound tenderness of the abdomen point to a pulmonary process rather than an intra-abdominal one.

Lab Data
Hematocrit

Anemia may be present with chronic bleeding.

White blood cell count

Normal is 5-10,000; an increase indicates infection. With appendicitis, about ½ of patients have a WBC over 10,000; however, a normal count is common. Usually there is a relative increase in the percentage of immature granulocytes. A WBC up to 25,000 may indicate ruptured appendix, abscess or peritonitis.

Differential

Neutrophils (60-70 %) are usually increased in bacterial infections; possibly with an increase in immature forms—bands.

Eosinophils (0-5 %) have a role in allergic conditions.

Lymphocytes (30-40 %) are increased in viral infections.

An increase in the neutrophil vs. lymphocyte ratio indicates bacterial infection.

Sickle cell prep

Positive with sickle cell disease. Abdominal pain is due to small thromboses in the viscera that result from aggregation of sickled cells.

Urinalysis

Indicated to rule out a urinary tract infection. Can also detect renal involvement (presence of casts), possible calculi (crystals), infectious process (bacteria, increased WBC) and bleeding (RBC). A metabolic imbalance may be detected with increased glucose or ketones. Increased bilirubin may be present with hepatic disease. Pregnancy test may be indicated.

Vaginal/urethral discharge

Gram stain of discharge can detect gonorrhea in males; a culture is needed in females. Wet prep may be indicated to diagnose vaginitis. See Vaginitis Protocol.

Liver function tests

Bilirubin, SGOT and SGPT are usually elevated with hepatic involvement. Alkaline phosphatase is increased if the common bile duct is obstructed. If SGOT and SGPT are normal and alkaline phosphatase is elevated, this indicates extrahepatic obstruction.

Enzymes

Amylase is elevated with acute pancreatitis within 24-48 hours. It is also increased with peptic ulcer perforation and obstruction of the small bowel. Urine amylase may be elevated without elevation in serum.

Lipase is elevated with acute pancreatitis, usually within 72-96 hours. It returns to normal more slowly than amylase. A lesser elevation may occur with carcinoma of the pancreas, tumors of the liver, cirrhosis of the liver, hepatitis and peritonitis.

Erythrocyte sedimentation rate (ESR)

Nonspecific test. A rough index of the presence of an inflammatory disease.

X-Rays
  Abdominal: flat and upright

Can detect free air, air in bowel, calcification and obstruction.

  Chest

Can help rule out respiratory pathology, cardiomegaly or abnormal aorta. Air under diaphragm is often seen better on chest x-ray than on abdominal film.

Electrocardiogram (EKG)

Changes in EKG may indicate cardiovascular origin of pain, e.g. myocardial infarction. Ischemic changes can be seen with some primary abdominal problems.

ASSESSMENT:

When making an assessment about the chief complaint of abdominal pain one must:

1. Determine whether or not the origin of the pain is an extra-abdominal condition which can mimic intra-abdominal conditions. For instance, diaphragmatic pleurisy, myocardial infarction or dissecting aneurysm.
2. Determine whether or not the origin of the pain is an acute pathologic process classified as "acute abdomen." There are six basic syndromes suggesting specific acute pathologic processes which cannot be missed. These are:

Inflammation

Gradual onset of pain; nausea and vomiting may be present. Tenderness is localized if the infectious process is localized, and diffuse tenderness and rigidity is present with an increased area of involvement as in peritonitis. Leukocytosis is present as is a slight fever. Examples of inflammation are: appendicitis, pancreatitis, cholecystitis.

Hemorrhage

Findings of peritonitis may be present along with local signs of blood loss in the peritoneal cavity. Fluid wave or shifting dullness may be present. Vital signs reflect blood loss. Purpura of umbilical, lumbar and inguinal areas may be present. These findings would be present with any intra- or retroperitoneal hemorrhage. One needs also to be alert to bleeding in the GI tract itself.

Obstruction

Colicky pain is often present. With small bowel obstruction there is a history of nausea and vomiting, constipation and abdominal distention. Bowel sounds, in small bowel obstruction, are increased with cramps. With large bowel obstruction, constipation and distention are present; bowel sounds may be normal and vomiting is not always present.

Perforation

There is an acute onset of pain which may subside but recurs later. Nausea and vomiting may be present at first, then subside only to return later. Bowel sounds may disappear; tenderness and rigidity are present. The patient is pale and sweaty, and has a weak pulse and shallow respirations. An example of a perforation is perforated peptic ulcer. Ruptured organs also present with sudden pain or signs of shock such as in ruptured ectopic pregnancy.

Ischemia

There is sudden onset of steady, severe pain. Nausea, vomiting, abdominal tenderness and decreased bowel sounds (with peritoneal involvement) are present. Shock is present with gangrene. Example: mesenteric artery occlusion.

Trauma

With a compatible history or any physical signs of trauma, any of the above processes may be present. Generally, with trauma of a solid viscus, signs of hemorrhage will be present, as with ruptured spleen. Trauma to hollow viscera (bowel) will present as peritonitis. There is shock with either.

3. If it is determined that an acute process is not the basis for the abdominal pain, then one can consider other less serious but more common causes for the pain. Examples of more commonly seen causes are:

Gastroenteritis	Associated with diarrhea, fever, nausea, vomiting and generalized arthralgias. Cause is often viral, with a duration of 24 hours to 3 days. Pain may be constant or intermittent cramping.
Peptic disease	Pain is usually a burning or gnawing sensation in the epigastric area. The most classic symptom is pain-eat-relief series of events. Nausea and vomiting may be present. The pain may also be precipitated by stress.
Hiatal hernia Esophageal reflux	Pain is midsternal, burning sensation occurring after meals. Regurgitation may also occur. Patient often states it feels like "heartburn" which may be relieved by antacids. May occur when bending or lying down, often awakening the patient at night.
Esophagitis	Pain is a midsternal, burning sensation.

PLAN:

Consultation/admission

A surgical consult is required for "acute abdomen." The treatment for acute situations is often surgical, e.g. appendicitis, tubal pregnancy, perforated ulcer. If an acute situation is ruled out, the patient will need further studies. Hospitalization is needed for acute situations requiring surgery as well as for medical conditions such as myocardial infarction or respiratory problems. It is also safer to hospitalize a patient if the diagnosis is in doubt.

Diagnostic
X-Rays

Further studies may be indicated to rule out pathology of specific areas of the gastrointestinal tract, e.g. upper gastrointestinal series, barium enema, gallbladder series. Intravenous pyelogram may be indicated if the urinary tract is suspected as origin of pain.

Sigmoidoscopy

In addition to the 40 % of cancer that can be palpated with rectal exam, another 30 % of colon cancer can be visualized with sigmoidoscopy.

Cultures

To rule out an infectious process:

Stool: rule out Shigella, Salmonella, Giardia and other parasites.

Urine: rule out urinary tract infection.

Gonorrhea: rule out gonorrhea. Must be done on selective media.

Bloods	See Liver Function Tests.
Therapeutic Antiemetic medications	For nausea and vomiting.
Analgesics	Antacids between meals have shown evidence of relieving pain of esophageal and ulcer origin. Choose an antacid according to other symptoms; e.g. magnesium will cause diarrhea, aluminum hydroxide will cause constipation. Various mixtures of the two are also available.
	Anticholinergics may help relieve pain of intestinal spasm. Use carefully as side effects include precipitating glaucoma, dry mouth and urinary retention. It is thought by some that unless side effects such as dry mouth occur, the treatment is ineffective.
Laxative or stool softeners	For constipation.
Antidiarrheics	Medications which decrease bowel motility as indicated.
Tranquilizers	May be used to help relieve tension. Counseling is in order also.
Diet	Liquid diet or frequent, small meals may be indicated to help reduce gastric motility and irritation, and to help neutralize acidity.
	Other treatment depends on further findings from diagnostic studies.
Patient education	In addition to sharing with the patient: 1) What is causing the pain (if

known), 2) What tests are to be done and 3) Expected outcome of treatment, other general areas for education are:

1. Education on use of medications and their side effects.
2. Diet instructions.
3. Importance of rest, physical and emotional.
4. Discontinuance of gastric irritants.
5. Reduction of risk factors.
6. Awareness of stressful situations which may affect the problem. Counseling to help patient modify his life-style is necessary.
7. When to return for follow-up and where (including referrals).
8. Specific information regarding why tests are to be done and the results.

BIBLIOGRAPHY

Aspects of Abdominal Pain, Nutley, New Jersey: Roche Laboratories, Division of Hoffman-LaRoche Inc., 1968.

Conn, Howard F., and Rex B. Conn, Jr., (eds.): *Current Diagnosis 4*, Philadelphia: Saunders, 1974.

DeGowin, Elmer L., and Richard L. DeGowin: *Bedside Diagnostic Examination*, New York: Macmillan, 1969.

MacBryde, C. M. (ed.): *Signs and Symptoms*, 5th ed., Philadelphia: Lippincott, 1970.

"Physical Examination of the Abdomen," *G.I. Series*, Parts 1-6, Richmond, Virginia: A. H. Robbins, 1974.

Sleisenger, Marvin H., and John S. Fordtran: *Gastrointestinal Disease*, Philadelphia: Saunders, 1973.

NOTES

60

NOTES

Chapter 5

Chest
pain

CHEST PAIN WORKSHEET

To be used in patients with:
Chest Pain

> *What you can't afford to miss: pulmonary embolism and infarction, pneumothorax, acute myocardial infarction, preinfarction angina, pneumonia, aortic dissection, pericarditis with effusion or tamponade.*

Chief Complaint:_____

SUBJECTIVE DATA:

Onset: _____Sudden _____Gradual _____Date

Location: _____

Frequency: _____

Duration: _____

Quality: _____

Severity at worst: _____

Radiation: _____

Precipitating/aggravating factors (e.g. exercise, meals, cold

weather, emotional upset, cough):_____

_____

Recent strenuous activity:_____

Relieving factors (if any): _____

History of trauma: _____

DESCRIBE POSITIVE RESPONSES
(Include Onset, Severity, Duration)

ASSOCIATED SYMPTOMS:
Yes   No

___ ___ Cough:

_____Nonproductive

_____Productive

_____Color: _____

_____Consistency: _____

_____Amount: _____

_____Hemoptysis: _____

___ ___ Fever/chills: _____

___ ___ Diaphoresis: _____

___ ___ Dyspnea/SOB: _____

___ ___ Nausea/vomiting: _____

___ ___ Numbness–tingling of extremities: _____

___ ___ Palpitations: _____

Protocols for Common Acute Self-Limiting Problems

___ ___ Flatulence/belching/bloating: _____

___ ___ Joint pain, stiffness:_____

___ ___ Other: _____

PAST MEDICAL HISTORY:
Yes *No*

___ ___ Previous similar episodes:

_____Number

_____Dates

_____Assessment

_____Treatment

___ ___ Medical or surgical illnesses (especially diabetes, obesity,

hypertension, hyperlipidemia): _____

_____

___ ___ Recent chest x-ray:

_____Date

_____Results

___ ___ Recent electrocardiogram:

_____Date

_____Results

___ ___ Current medications: _____

___ ___ Significant family history:_____

___ ___ Habits:

     _____Smoking

     _____Alcohol

___ ___ Occupational risk: _____

OBJECTIVE DATA:
    Vital signs: _____B/P _____P (rate and rhythm)

          _____R _____T _____Wt

    General appearance: _____

DESCRIBE POSITIVE RESPONSES

CHEST EXAM: _____Not Done
Yes   *No*

___ ___ Cyanosis:_____

___ ___ Deformity or abnormal contour:_____

___ ___ Asymmetrical expansion: _____

___ ___ Thoracic spine deformity:_____

___ ___ Skin lesions: _____

___ ___ Dullness:

          _____Location

___ ___ Fremitus (increased/decreased):

          _____Tactile

          _____Vocal

Protocols for Common Acute Self-Limiting Problems

___ ___ Tenderness (include spine): _____

___ ___ Restricted movement of diaphragm:_____

___ ___ Abnormal breath sounds (rales, rhonchi, wheezes): ___

___ ___ Friction rub: _____

___ ___ E to A changes:_____

NECK EXAM: _____Not Done
Yes *No*

___ ___ Tracheal shift: _____

___ ___ Jugular venous distention: _____

___ ___ Carotid bruits/diminished quality of pulse: _____

___ ___ Lymphadenopathy (describe location, size, number,

        texture, movability, tenderness): _____

        _____

___ ___ Cervical spine deformity/tenderness: _____

___ ___ Paraspinous muscle spasm: _____

BREAST EXAM: _____Not Done
Yes *No*

___ ___ Contour irregularities: _____

___ ___ Nipples (inversion/discharge): _____

___ ___ Tenderness: _____

___ ___ Masses:_____

___ ___ Axillary lymphadenopathy: _____

CARDIOVASCULAR EXAM: _____Not Done

Yes   *No*

____ ____ Irregular rhythm: _____

____ ____ Precordium abnormal:

            _____Point of maximum impulse

            Character of:

                              _____S-1

                              _____S-2

____ ____ Heaves/thrills: _____

____ ____ Extra sounds: _____

____ ____ Murmurs:_____

LEG EXAM: _____Not Done

Yes   *No*

____ ____ Tenderness: _____

____ ____ Swelling: _____

____ ____ Discoloration: _____

____ ____ Positive Homans's sign:_____

____ ____ Peripheral pulses unequal: _____

____ ____ Quality of pulse abnormal: _____

____ ____ Other: _____

SHOULDER EXAM: _____Not Done

Yes   *No*

____ ____ Tenderness: _____

___ ___ Erythema: _____

___ ___ Effusion: _____

___ ___ Stiffness: _____

___ ___ Limitation of range of motion: _____

___ ___ Crepitus: _____

ABDOMINAL EXAM: _____Not Done
Yes   No

___ ___ Scars, lesions: _____

___ ___ Percussion abnormal: _____

___ ___ Bowel sounds abnormal: _____

___ ___ Liver palpable: _____

___ ___ Spleen palpable: _____

___ ___ Tenderness: _____

___ ___ Masses:_____

LAB DATA:
Done Not
       Done

___ ___ CBC (differential):

          _____Results

___ ___ Erythrocyte sedimentation rate:_____

___ ___ Sputum:

          _____Gross exam

          _____Gram stain

___ ___ Urinalysis: _____

___ ___ Electrocardiogram: _____

___ ___ Chest x-ray:_____

___ ___ Rib films:_____

___ ___ Cervical spine films: _____

___ ___ Thoracic spine films: _____

___ ___ Arterial blood gases: _____

___ ___ Lung scan: _____

ASSESSMENT:

_____

_____

_____

_____

PLAN:

_____ Admit

_____ Diagnostic:

_____Viral serology/culture

_____Cold agglutinins

_____VDRL

_____Sputum culture

_____Tine test/PPD/other skin tests

_____Bronchoscopy

_____Bronchogram

_____Upper gastrointestinal series

_____Barium swallow

_____Oral cholecystogram

_____Treadmill test

_____Pulmonary function tests

_____Other diagnostic tests: _____

_____ Therapeutic (medications given, dosage, schedule and number dispensed):

_____Analgesic: _____

_____Antipyretic:_____

_____Antibiotic: _____

_____Antacids: _____

_____Cough suppressant/expectorant:_____

_____Bronchodilators: _____

_____Nitrates: _____

_____Other_____

_____ Patient Education:

_____Call for test results:_____

_____Date

_____Return to clinic date: _____

_____Criteria for return to clinic: _____

_____Medication usage: _____

_____Referral to other clinics: _____

_____Specific therapies (e.g. rest, local heat, humidifier,

vaporizer use): _____

_____

CHEST PAIN WORKSHEET RATIONALE

SUBJECTIVE DATA:

Onset

Helps differentiate acute vs. chronic process. Activity at or around the time of onset is often a clue to differentiating angina from other causes of chest pain.

Location

Unilateral or localized pain is often associated with trauma or inflammation. Pleuritic pain can be bilateral or unilateral (often posterior). Cardiac pain is often not well localized; bizarre distributions can be seen in cardiac neuroses. In one study of 150 cases of acute myocardial infarction, all patients had some anterior trunk pain.

Frequency

Peptic disease often flares in the spring or fall. Pain at night is seen with peptic disease, angina decubitus and hiatus hernia.

Duration

This correlates roughly with how long the noxious stimulus lasts:

Transient pain is often related to movement of injured ligaments or muscles.

Persistent, boring pain that is often worse at night is seen with bony erosion.

A steady pain, worse with movement, is seen with musculoskeletal origin.

Angina lasts several minutes or less.

The pain of myocardial infarction, biliary disease and renal colic can last for hours.

Quality

The intensity of the pain generally varies with the intensity of the stimulus. The response can be blocked by drugs or distraction, or augmented by fear. The patient should describe the quality of pain in his own words. Examples:

Skin: pricking, itching pain.

Esophageal: burning.

Cardiac ischemia: heavy, crushing, gripping, squeezing, tight and occasionally burning or searing.

Musculoskeletal: dull, aching.

Peptic disease: gnawing, burning, hungry sensation.

Cholecystitis: bloating, distention.

Dissecting aneurysm: tearing.

Nerve root: sharp, shooting, transient.

Severity at Worst

This is subject to variation. It is important to remember that the severity of the pain may not correlate with the seriousness of the illness.

Radiation

The pattern of radiation is subject to variation and is not always an indicator of the responsible body segment. For example, pain in the neck, arms or jaw can be secondary to myocardial ischemia.

Precipitating/Aggravating Factors
  Recent strenuous activity
  History of trauma

A relation of pain to the intake of food can sometimes help distinguish gastrointestinal from cardiac causes of chest pain (see discussion on p. 82 for classic precipitating factors of angina pectoris). Recent activity or trauma may be helpful in diagnosing musculoskeletal pain.

Relieving Factors

The pain of peptic disease may be relieved by food or alkali. Common analgesics, rest or immobilization may help in skeletal, muscular and ligamentous disorders. Rest and nitroglycerin usually relieve the pain of angina, although nitroglycerin can occasionally relieve spasm of the gastrointestinal tract.

Associated Symptoms
  Cough

Is present with tracheobronchitis, pneumonia, tumors, pulmonary embolism and tuberculosis.

  Hemoptysis

Hemoptysis may be seen with any of these but its presence requires detailed investigation.

Fever/chills

Classically seen with infection, but can be seen with some tumors, especially of the mediastinum.

Diaphoresis

May be seen with any severe pain or castastrophic event such as myocardial infarction, pulmonary embolism or dissecting aneurysm. Also seen with tumors and infections.

Dyspnea/shortness of breath

Seen with pneumonia, myocardial infarction, pulmonary embolism, tuberculosis and tumors.

Nausea/vomiting

Can be associated with myocardial ischemia or infarction and with gastrointestinal disorders.

Numbness/tingling of extremities

Can occur with ischemic heart disease; also seen with hyperventilation which may be associated with perioral tingling.

Palpitations

May be associated with arrhythmias such as paroxysmal atrial tachycardia and premature ventricular contractions. These may be normal or associated with myocardial infarction.

Flatulence/belching/ bloating

Often associated with gallbladder disease.

Joint pain/stiffness

Associated with bursitis, arthritis and tendonitis. These conditions may refer pain to the thoracic area.

Past Medical History
Previous similar episodes

Many of the causes of chest pain (e.g. angina) may lead to recurrent episodes.

Medical/surgical illnesses

Diabetes, hypertension, hyperlipidemia and obesity are associated with an increased risk of arteriosclerotic cardiovascular disease. A history of any serious past illness may affect your diagnostic and therapeutic plan.

Recent chest x-ray
EKG

If the results of these are known or available, they may provide help in reaching the correct diagnosis.

Family history

A family history of respiratory or cardiovascular disease can be useful in evaluating the patient's complaint. This includes a family history of early myocardial infarct or sudden death.

Habits
Occupational risk

Smoking, alcohol use and occupation give information about the patient's life style which may help in evaluating the relative risk for cardiovascular disease. For example, there is increased risk with heavy smoking and sedentary or stressful occupations.

OBJECTIVE DATA:
Vital signs

Temperature and pulse are increased with infection, inflammation and some systemic disease. A low-grade fever can be seen several days after an acute myocardial infarct.

Hypertension may be associated with cardiovascular disease.

Rate and depth of respiration may be altered with pneumothorax, anxiety, diaphragmatic disease (subphrenic abscess) or central nervous system lesions.

Sighing respirations are often seen in anxious and depressed persons.

Chest Exam
Inspection
Cyanosis
Deformity
Asymmetry
Skin lesions

You may see labored breathing and use of accessory muscles with respiratory distress and chronic obstructive pulmonary disease. Look for cyanosis which may be central and/or peripheral. Look for deformities, scars due to previous surgery, evidence of trauma; pectus excavatum is rarely associated with chest pain.

Chest expansion may be limited by ankylosing spondylitis, pleuritic pain, pneumothorax, pleural effusion, pneumonia or fractured ribs.

Symmetry may be altered by kyphosis, scoliosis or localized swellings.

Observe for frequency and effectiveness of cough.

Skin may show the vesicular lesions of herpes zoster, ecchymoses (trauma), or the pallor associated with anemia, shock and chronic disease.

Percussion
Dullness

This is decreased in atelectasis, pneumonia, pleural effusion, thickened pleura and mass lesions. Increased resonance is seen in emphysema and pneumothorax.

Palpation
Fremitus

Tactile fremitus is decreased or absent in pleural effusion, thickened pleura or pneumothorax; it may be increased with consolidation.

Tenderness
Tenderness and spasm is found in muscle strain, local trauma, injuries to the vertebrae and local inflammation such as skin infection or abscess.

Restricted movement
Excursion of diaphragm is limited with pleurisy and pleural effusions. Paradoxical motion and crepitus may occur with rib fracture.

Auscultation
Diminished breath sounds are due to decreased airflow or increased insulation as with fat or air. Breath sounds are decreased with chronic pulmonary disease, pneumothorax, shallow breathing and pleural effusions.

Abnormal breath sounds
  Rales
Fine or crepitant rales are associated with pneumonia, early congestive heart failure or interstitial pulmonary disease. Medium rales are associated with late pneumonia or pulmonary edema. Coarse rales can be heard in all of these conditions. Rales are thought to have their origin at the alveolar level and are due to opening of the alveoli.

Rhonchi
Caused by mucus or fluid rattling in the tracheobronchial tree.

Wheezes
Due to airway narrowing, usually from bronchospasm. Associated with asthma, foreign bodies and mucous plugging.

Friction rub	This is a grating sensation that is heard or palpated. The origin is inflamed pleural surfaces rubbing against each other.
E-A changes Whispered pectoriloquy	Found in consolidation with an open airway and with compressed, fluid-filled alveoli; also found in pleural effusions.

Neck Exam

Tracheal shift	Occurs with pneumothorax, pleural effusion or atelectasis.
Venous distention	Seen in congestive heart failure and superior vena cava obstruction.
Carotid bruits/ diminished pulse	May give an indication of generalized vascular disease.
Lymphadenopathy	May be an indication of local infection (viral or bacterial) or possibly of systemic disease.
Cervical spine deformity Muscle spasm	The cervical spine and muscle exam may uncover a local problem that is causing chest pain.

Breast Exam

Indications of breast disease include irregularities, dimpling, nipple retraction, peau d'orange appearance, edema, unusual pigmentation, ulcerations, discharges and masses. Any disease in the breast causing pain may be initially thought to be chest pain by the patient.

Cardiovascular Exam

Irregular rhythm	May be indicative of atrial fibrillation or premature ventricular contractions. PVC's are seen normally

as well as in acute myocardial infarction.

Palpation
Percussion

Determination of the point of maximal impulse and left border of cardiac dullness gives an indication of cardiac size, ventricular enlargement and possibly ventricular aneurysm. Thrills are felt with Grade IV or louder murmurs.

Auscultation
　Extra sounds
　Murmurs

Listen to quality of heart sounds; they are often diminished in acute infarction. Gallops may be heard with congestive failure; S_4 is common during myocardial ischemia. A soft systolic murmur at the apex may be indicative of papillary muscle dysfunction.

Leg Exam

You are looking for signs of peripheral vascular disease (cool, cyanotic leg with poor or absent distal pulses). Also look for signs of venous disease and thrombophlebitis which may point to pulmonary embolus as cause of chest pain (leg is swollen, red, hot and tender).

Shoulder Exam

Observe for pain on motion, tenderness and possibly heat that may be a sign of arthritis, bursitis or tendonitis.

Abdominal Exam

Many abdominal processes can cause chest pain or discomfort. See abdominal causes of chest pain under Assessment.

Lab Data
　Complete blood count
　(CBC)

This is useful to detect the presence of infection, other inflammation and anemia which may precipitate angina. Leukocytosis occurs with bacterial infection and sometimes 1-3 days after a myocardial infarction. Lymphocytosis with large atypical lymphs is seen with many viral infections.

Erythrocyte sedimentation rate (ESR)

This is a nonspecific indicator of inflammation. It may be increased in infections, neoplastic disease and collagen diseases. It also becomes elevated 2-3 days after an acute myocardial infarct, decreasing slowly to normal over the next month.

Sputum

Examination may help detect specific pathogens: gram stain for pneumonia, acid fast stain for tuberculosis and cytology for malignancy.

Urinalysis

Microscopic hematuria may be seen with dissecting aneurysm or bacterial endocarditis.

Electrocardiogram (EKG)

This is extremely useful in evaluation of cardiac disease, but it is to be remembered that a patient can have angina or early myocardial infarction and a normal EKG. Arrhythmias and electrolyte imbalance can also be detected or inferred.

Myocardial infarction when detected presents as ST segment elevation, with Q waves in the leads corresponding to the affected segment of myocardium.

Pulmonary embolus may cause atrial arrhythmias or right axis deviation.

Chest x-ray	This is useful in detecting infiltrates, effusions, lobar consolidation, segmental infarction (wedge-shaped infiltrate), masses, rib fractures and cardiomegaly.
Cervical/thoracic spine x-ray	Can detect fracture, arthritis and other bony deformities.
Arterial blood gases	A decrease in arterial partial pressure of oxygen may be seen in pulmonary embolus and pneumonia.
Lung scan	This is useful, if easily available, in ruling out pulmonary embolus. Classically, a defect in circulation is seen with normal ventilation and a normal chest x-ray.
ASSESSMENT:	This consists of trying to correlate the historical and physical findings with one of the categories listed below. Often it is not possible to confidently assess the problem according to the following classification. The most likely etiology or etiologies for the pain should be decided and further tests scheduled to clarify the diagnosis.

Cardiac Causes of Chest Pain

Pericardial pain	This is substernal or just to the left of the sternum and may increase with swallowing, deep inspiration, torsion of trunk, sitting up or rolling from side to side. It is a sharp, stabbing, intermittent or continuous pain. It can resemble the pain of myocardial infarction and is associated with fever, malaise, increased erythrocyte sedimentation

rate and leukocytosis. Findings include a pericardial friction rub (from friction of surfaces of two pericardial membranes), electrocardiographic changes and x-ray changes which show increased size of cardiac shadow due to the presence of pericardial fluid; 25-50 % have concurrent pleural effusions.

Angina pectoris

This is usually a substernal, visceral pain or heaviness, provoked by emotion, effort, eating, cold weather, tobacco and occasionally by lying down. It sometimes occurs in the morning shortly after arising, while shaving, etc. It is of moderate intensity. Never stabbing, never increased by cough or movements. It may radiate to the arms, neck or jaw, often as an aching, vague discomfort accompanied by numbness and tingling. A fourth heart sound may be heard. The lungs are clear. The electrocardiogram may be normal or show evidence of ischemic heart disease (ST segment depression, previous myocardial infarct). Blood pressure is normal or elevated. There are no specific laboratory findings. The pain is relieved in minutes by rest or sublingual nitroglycerin. Intermediate syndromes between angina pectoris and acute myocardial infarction are called preinfarction angina, unstable angina and crescendo angina. Pain tends to be precipitated by less effort, occurs more frequently and lasts longer. It is a change in the patient's previous pattern of angina and requires hospitalization.

Myocardial infarction

The pain is similar to that of angina but more severe and prolonged, crushing, gripping and "indescribable." The radiation is similar to that of angina. It can continue for hours, sometimes controlled only by morphine. Nausea, vomiting and hypertension are not uncommon. Electrocardiographic changes (elevated ST segment, Q waves, arrhythmias) and laboratory changes (increased transaminase, sedimentation rate, leukocytosis) may not be present on the initial presentation. Pain referred to the abdomen can resemble pancreatitis, perforation and other acute abdominal conditions. This is confusing especially when leukocytosis is present. Treatment consists of immediate hospitalization and control of pain and accompanying symptoms and complications (shock, cardiac failure, arrhythmias). Infarction can be followed immediately or months later by painful disability of shoulder and hands ("shoulder-hand syndrome").

Aortic pain

This may be due to inflammation, dilatation, dissection or rupture. The pain of dissecting aneurysm is sudden, severe, agonizing, "tearing," substernal or diffuse over the upper anterior chest and shoulders. As the dissection proceeds over the arch it involves pain in neck and back, especially the interscapular area. Rarely the pain is mild. Dissection usually occurs in patients with pre-existing arterial hypertension. Syphilitic aortitis or aneurysm is often painless and dissection is rare.

Pleuropulmonary Causes of Chest Pain

Pleurisy/pleuritis

Can be secondary to infections, infarction, neoplasm. It is seen sometimes with liver abscess and systemic diseases such as systemic lupus erythematosus. It is characterized by dyspnea and chest pain on inspiration usually over the lower half of the thorax, and may be referred to the upper abdomen and along the costal margins. Neck and shoulder pain can be present with diaphragmatic pleurisy with effusion. Physical signs include dependent dullness to percussion, distant or absent breath sounds and fremitus and decreased excursion on the affected side. Treatment consists in identifying and treating the underlying cause. Analgesics and anti-inflammatory agents may be useful.

Epidemic pleurodynia

Often presents with the abrupt onset of severe pleuritic pain along the costal margins or in the shoulder girdle. It is caused by a Coxsackie virus. Occasionally one may find basilar rales and dullness due to effusion. Course is 2-7 days. Treatment is bed rest and analgesia.

Pulmonary infarction and embolism

Embolism is more common with medical conditions than after surgical procedures; more common in people over 40 years of age and those with prolonged bed rest or immobilization. Many cases go undiagnosed. Small emboli cause transient mild symptoms such as fever, episodic weakness, transient dyspnea and tachycardia, sometimes with little chest pain, though classically sudden chest pain, anxiety, dyspnea and hemoptysis may occur. Electrocardiographic changes are uncommon. Physical findings may include signs of consolidation and an evident focus of peripheral venous thrombosis. Embolism can mimic other diseases including viral pneumonia and post-op atelectasis. With massive embolism, the picture may resemble that of acute myocardial infarction.

Pulmonary infections

Pain is present if the tracheobronchial tract is involved (mild substernal soreness or burning) or pleuritic pain may occur if the pleura is involved. Pneumonias are either bacterial (pneumococci, streptococci, staphylococci, klebsiella), viral (influenza A and B, rubella) or mycoplasmal.

Pulmonary tumors

The symptoms produced by cancer depend on the size of the lesion. Pain is rarely present in early stages and is usually vague. Persistent bronchopulmonary infections may mask underlying malignancy and should be followed with serial chest x-rays.

Primary tumor of the pleura

Rare. Most common is mesothelioma. There may be constant chest pain, cough and dyspnea.

Smoker's lung

This may be present as rhythmic darting anterior chest pains, chronic pharyngitis, wheezing and dyspnea with frequent respiratory infections which progress to chronic bronchitis. Sometimes disappears with cessation of smoking.

Other Intrathoracic
Causes of Chest Pain

Diaphragmatic pain

Diaphragmatic hernia pain is similar to mild epigastric distress or peptic disease. Sometimes it is referred to the lower sternum with subphrenic abscess and there may be tenderness to palpation along costal margins with marked inspiratory pain. A "stitch" or side ache is associated with strenuous exercise and is probably secondary to diaphragmatic or intercostal spasm or ischemia.

Large mediastinal tumors

Can exist without pain or other bothersome symptoms. Pain when it is present is usually associated with dyspnea, cough and a gradually increasing sensation of weight on the sternum.

Mediastinitis

Can be caused by 1) trauma (gunshot or stab wounds and perforation of the esophagus by foreign bodies or instruments); 2) infection of contiguous structures and 3) infection of lung (empyema, abscess) or neck. Pain can be mild and nebulous or there can be pain with inspiration or swallowing.

Esophagitis

Can simulate or be indistinguishable from cardiac pain. Dysphagia is the most common manifestation of esophageal disease which can be inflammatory, obstructive, neurogenic or secondary to systemic disease such as scleroderma. Other common manifestations of esophageal disease include: excessive salivation, gurgling sounds when swallowing, regurgitation (especially of undigested food), coughing after drinking liquids, hoarseness and ultimately weight loss. Esophagitis is the most common esophageal disease and is usually found in older people with hiatal hernia and esophageal ulcerations; it is also found with frequent vomiting in early pregnancy, in pyloric obstruction, duodenal ulcer, chronic gastritis and with esophageal diverticula (Zenker's diverticulum). Gastric acid reflux with erosion is the direct cause of esophagitis. Esophageal pain is deep, central, burning, substernal and occasionally radiates to the shoulders. It may have a nocturnal occurrence when the patient is lying down. It may be relieved by food, antacids and the upright position. Treatment consists of elevating the head of the bed, weight reduction, no tight clothes and antacids. Surgery may be indicated to correct hiatus hernia.

Cardiospasm

Seen in the 4th decade of life. Physiologic obstruction at the distal esophageal junction with proximal dilatation of the esophagus results in spasm of the entire esophagus. This can result in constant dysphagia and substernal distress. Spasm is seen on fluoroscopy along with dilatation. Liquids are often regurgitated while solids can be swallowed. Treatment consists of antispasmodics to relax the distal esophageal sphincter, and mild sedation.

Abdominal Causes of Chest Pain

Abdominal problems

Abdominal conditions causing pain in the chest include gallbladder disease, acute and chronic pancreatitis, carcinoma, cysts of the pancreas, peptic esophagitis and ulcer, aerophagia, carcinoma of the stomach, gastric diverticula, colon flexure syndromes, carcinoid tumor and rupture and infarction of the spleen. Subdiaphragmatic conditions and their complications present characteristic patterns of pain. A careful history and physical exam with appropriate tests can help to establish a diagnosis. See Abdominal Pain Protocol.

The following conditions may cause chest wall pain arising from:

Skin

Herpes zoster

Is an acute viral disease that is more severe and prolonged in older patients. A prodrome of 3-4 days usually with fever and malaise is common. It is characterized by clusters of vesicular lesions along intercostal nerve distributions. The pain is burning and there is often hyperalgesia.

Intercostal nerve pain

Is due to irritation of or pressure on an intercostal nerve. It is of sudden onset, localized, aggravated by cold, inspiration, cough and movements of the upper torso. Its quality is stabbing or burning.

Breast
  Nonspecific breast pain

Can be seen cyclically after hysterectomy and premenstrually. Either or both breasts can be affected. It is due to vascular engorgement and sodium retention. The glandular nature of the breast is subject to endocrine influences. Chlorothiazide and ammonium chloride have been helpful in some cases.

  Cystic disease

Causes pain and tenderness to palpation continuously or only premenstrually. Aspiration of cyst contents gives relief.

  Mondor's disease

Is seen most often in women with pendulous breasts. It is a thrombophlebitis of the superficial veins of the breast and anterior chest wall (especially thoracoepigastric vein). It usually follows minor trauma or breast surgery and subsides spontaneously.

Muscle
  Trauma

With strains, sprains, direct injury and hematoma, the muscular pain and tenderness is limited to distribution of the affected muscle. Causes of diffuse myalgias include systemic infections, strenuous exercise, incessant cough and trichinosis. Treatment consists of heat, rest, mild analgesia and correction of the underlying cause.

Inflammatory

Myositis can be due to infections, allergies or unknown factors. The responsible agent is often not identified. The cause can be bacterial (tuberculosis), viral (Coxsackie) or parasitic (trichinosis). It can be related to systemic illnesses like polymyositis, dermatomyositis, rheumatic fever, scleroderma, systemic lupus erythematosus and polyarteritis.

Skeletal

The shoulder joint, although at the periphery of the chest, is often the site of pain that can arise from any individual unit of the shoulder joint.

Bursitis

Is often acute, with sudden onset of pain which increases quickly in intensity causing complete restriction of movement of the joint and upper arm. It can be brought on by slight trauma or strain. It may become subacute or chronic with tenderness over the greater tuberosity of the humerus and a catching pain with elevation or abduction of the arm.

Tendonitis

May be associated with chronic trauma (often occupational) and degeneration secondary to aging. Pain varies from a mild, nagging to a sharp, stabbing quality. Most common sites are the supraspinatus, infraspinatus, teres minor and subscapularis tendons. Other causes of shoulder pain include osteoarthritis, acute rheumatic fever, tuberculosis, infections (gonorrhea, brucellosis), Reiter's syndrome, gouty arthritis, Paget's disease, trauma and rheumatoid arthritis.

Ostalgia

Diseases of the periosteum present with intense, well-localized pain. Trauma may cause periostitis and acute osteomyelitis. The pain is sharp, severe and continuous. Malignant metastases to the thoracic vertebrae produce intense, aching, boring pain, usually worse at night.

The pain of *rib fracture* increases with breathing, coughing, sneezing and bending. There is often tenderness and swelling at the site of fracture and there may be local crepitus. The treatment of the uncomplicated fracture consists of analgesia (oral or local., e.g. nerve block). Strapping helps symptoms by decreasing respiratory movements but may lead to atelectasis and pneumonia.

Tietze's syndrome
(costochondritis)

The cause is unknown. It is characterized by an ill-defined pain with localized tenderness with or without swelling at one or more costochondral or chondrosternal junctions; sometimes associated with a history of injury. It more commonly affects the upper ribs. Treatment consists of reassurance, heat and analgesia; use of oral corticosteroids may prevent recurrences.

Pain from cervical spines

Extrusion of intervertebral disc causes root compression and dorsal root pain from irritation of dorsal nerve radicles. This is referred along a peripheral nerve course. The pain is intermittent, sharp and stabbing and follows a nerve root distribution.

Bone tumors and infections (staphylococcal, tuberculous, Salmonella)	May cause bone pain by local invasion, extension and irritation of the periosteum.

PLAN:
Diagnostic

Viral serology/culture	Appropriate swabs with acute and convalescent sera can be sent to the hospital or most state laboratories for viral isolation.
Cold agglutinins	Useful in identifying or suggesting a mycoplasmal etiology to the illness.
VDRL	Coupled with the FTA-ABS test for syphilis, this is useful in helping diagnose syphilitic aortitis. The VDRL may be falsely positive in lupus erythematosus.
Sputum culture	May identify specific bacterial or mycobacterial (tuberculosis) pathogens.
Tine test/PPD Other skin tests	Useful in diagnosing tuberculosis, histoplasmosis, coccidioidomycosis.
Bronchoscopy	Used to directly visualize an endobronchial lesion.
Bronchogram	Useful in diagnosing distal endobronchial lesions and bronchiectasis.
Upper gastrointestinal series Barium swallow	This is useful in ruling out esophageal and other upper gastrointestinal tract causes of chest pain.
Oral cholecystogram	To rule out gallbladder disease.

Treadmill test	This is an electrocardiogram recorded during graded exercise and is useful in documenting myocardial ischemia if ST segment depression occurs.
Pulmonary function tests	These will document the degree of pulmonary disease present but do not point to a specific cause for chest pain.
Therapeutic	See treatment for specific conditions under Assessment.
Patient education	Chest pain can be a frightening occurrence and the patient will require support and reassurance. A careful explanation of appropriate data, further studies and specifics of the therapeutic program will do much to allay anxiety and encourage compliance.

BIBLIOGRAPHY

Harrison, T. R., and T. J. Reeves: *Principles and Problems of Ischemic Heart Disease*, Chicago: Year Book Medical Publishers, 1968.

Harvey, A. M., et al. (eds.): *The Principles and Practice of Medicine*, 18th ed., New York: Appleton-Century-Crofts, 1972.

Hurst, J. W., and R. B. Logue: *The Heart, Arteries and Veins*, 2nd ed., New York: McGraw Hill, 1970.

Knapp, Marcus A., and M. J. Chatton: *Current Diagnosis and Treatment*, Los Altos, California: Lange Medical Publishers, 1972.

MacBryde, C. B. (ed.): *Signs and Symptoms*, 5th ed., Philadelphia: Lippincott, 1970.

Wehrmacher, W. H.: *Pain in the Chest*, Springfield, Illinois: Charles C Thomas, 1964.

Wintrobe, M. W., et al. (eds.): *Harrison's Principles of Internal Medicine*, 7th ed., New York: McGraw Hill, 1974.

NOTES

Chapter 6

Diarrhea

DIARRHEA WORKSHEET

To be used in patients with:
Loose Stools
Bloody Stools
Stools at Night
Abdominal Cramps with Stools

What you can't afford to miss: diarrhea associated with gastrointestinal hemorrhage, ulcerative colitis and toxic megacolon, mesenteric infarction, bowel obstruction, severe dehydration.

Chief Complaint:_____

SUBJECTIVE DATA:

Onset: _____Sudden _____Gradual

Duration: _____Days _____Weeks _____Months

Character of stools:

Volume in 24 hours: _____

Frequency: _____

Consistency:

_____Liquid

_____Soft

_____Foamy, floating

Appearance:

_____Color: _____

_____Gross blood

_____Oil

_____Mucus

_____Pus/exudate

_____Undigested food

Time:

_____Day only:_____

_____Day/night: _____

_____After meals: _____

Course:

_____Progressive: _____

_____Intermittent: _____

_____Resolving: _____

_____Stable/unchanged: _____

Describe Positive Responses
(Include Onset, Severity, Duration, Location)

PRECIPATED BY:

Yes   *No*

____ ____ Medications: _____

____ ____ Stress/environmental changes: _____

____ ____ Foods: _____

____ ____ Activity: _____

____ ____ Unusual water source: _____

____ ____ Other_____

RELIEVED BY:

Yes   *No*

____ ____ Medication:_____

____ ____ Fasting: _____

____ ____ Decreased stress: _____

____ ____ Nothing _____

            Therapy tried: _____

____ ____ Other_____

ASSOCIATED WITH:

Yes   *No*

____ ____ Cramping/abdominal pain: _____

____ ____ Urgency/tenesmus: _____

____ ____ Fever/chills/sweats:_____

____ ____ Nausea/vomiting: _____

____ ____ Weakness/hot flashes:_____

____ ____ Intermittent constipation:_____

____ ____ Weight loss: _____

____ ____ Travel exposure: _____

____ ____ Family/associates with same: _____

____ ____ Ingestion of particular meal: _____

PAST MEDICAL HISTORY:
Yes   No

____ ____ History of diarrhea:_____

____ ____ Other illnesses associated with diarrhea: _____

____ ____ Other gastrointestinal diseases: _____

____ ____ Past abdominal surgeries:_____

Complications: _____

____ ____ Previous hospitalizations:_____

____ ____ Medications: _____

OBJECTIVE DATA:
Vital signs: _____B/P _____P _____R _____T _____Wt

ABDOMINAL EXAM: _____Not Done
Yes   No

____ ____ Scars, skin turgor:_____

____ ____ Asymmetry:_____

____ ____ Abnormal bulging/distention: _____

____ ____ Visible peristaltic waves: _____

___ ___ Abnormal bowel sounds: _____

___ ___ Friction rubs:_____

___ ___ Bruits: _____

___ ___ Mass:_____

___ ___ Liver palpable: _____

___ ___ Spleen palpable: _____

___ ___ Tenderness/rebound: _____

___ ___ Rigidity: _____

___ ___ Fluid wave: _____

___ ___ Percussed resonance:_____

___ ___ Shifting dullness:_____

RECTAL EXAM: _____Not Done
Yes   No

___ ___ External hemorrhoids: _____

___ ___ Fistula/abscess:_____

___ ___ Sphincter tone abnormal: _____

___ ___ Tenderness: _____

___ ___ Mass:_____

___ ___ Impaction: _____

GENERAL EXAM: _____Not Done
Yes   No

___ ___ Inappropriate affect: _____

___ ___ Dehydrated: _____

___ ___ Increased pigmentation: _____

___ ___ Weight loss/evidence:_____

___ ___ Thyroid disease:

_____Thyroid palpable:_____

_____Exophthalmos: _____

_____Fine tremor: _____

_____Tachycardia: _____

_____Lid lag:_____

___ ___ Lymphadenopathy: _____

___ ___ Neurologic exam:

Peripheral reflexes:_____

Sensation: _____

LAB DATA:
STOOL EXAM: _____Not Done
Done Not
**   Done**

___ ___ Gross: Blood_____Pus_____Mucus_____

Oil_____Undigested meat fiber_____

___ ___ Hematest:

_____Positive

_____Negative

___ ___ Microscopic:

_____Ova

_____Parasite

_____RBC

_____WBC

____ ____ Odor:

        _____Normal

        _____Foul

____ ____ Sudan stain:

        _____Positive

        _____Negative

OTHER LAB:_____Not Done

____ ____ CBC with differential: _____

____ ____ Electrolytes/BUN: _____

____ ____ Urinalysis: _____Specific gravity _____Sugar

        _____Bilirubin

____ ____ Radiology (3 way of abdomen): _____

ASSESSMENT:

_____

_____

_____

_____

PLAN:
DIAGNOSTIC:

_____ Stool

       _____Ova and parasites

       _____Culture and sensitivity

_____ Bloods

       _____CBC with differential

       _____Electrolytes/BUN

       _____Glucose

       _____T_3/T_4

_____ Sigmoidoscopy

       Date:_____

_____ Barium enema

_____ UGI with small bowel follow-through

_____ 72 hour stool for fat

       Dates:_____

THERAPEUTIC:

_____ Consultation: _____

_____ Rest: _____

_____ Diet: _____

_____ Removal of causative factors: _____

_____ Drugs (give dose, schedule and amount dispensed)

_____Kaolin-pectin (Kaopectate): _____

_____Anticholinergic: _____

_____Diphenoxylate (Lomotil): _____

_____Opiates: _____

_____Antibiotic: _____

_____Other: _____

PATIENT EDUCATION:

_____ Return if worse or not better in_____days:_____

_____ Call for test results: _____

_____ Stool isolation precautions: _____

_____ Return for follow-up: _____

_____ Appointment to another clinic: _____

_____ Other:_____

DIARRHEA WORKSHEET RATIONALE

Diarrhea is defined as an alteration of bowel habits of the individual, specifically characterized by increased frequency and/or increased fluid consistency of the stools. This should be evaluated in terms of change from the patient's "normal" bowel habits. Most individuals have short, self-limited episodes of diarrhea infrequently throughout their lifetime without long-term significance.

The following are life-threatening disease processes with diarrhea which the practitioner cannot afford to miss on initial evaluation, and which require hospitalization.

1. Diarrhea associated with upper or lower gastrointestinal hemorrhage.
2. Severe ulcerative colitis with toxic megacolon.
3. Ischemic bowel disease with mesenteric infarction.

4. Partial to complete bowel obstruction.
5. Addison's disease with severe dehydration.
6. Severe dehydration.

A comprehensive history of illness, past and present, is necessary to establish the plan for determining the etiology. The following is information important in making an assessment and planning treatment.

SUBJECTIVE RATIONALE:
Onset
Sudden vs. gradual

Indicative of acute vs. chronic diarrhea, although chronic forms (e.g. ulcerative colitis) can present initially as an acute diarrhea.

Duration

Indicative of acute, possibly self-limiting vs. chronic disease.

Quality and Character of Stools
Volume in 24 hours

Large volumes indicative of secretory (cholera, *E. coli*) or malabsorption (small intestine) diarrhea.

Frequency

Frequent, small volumes with tenesmus indicative of inflammation of colon/rectal area such as with ulcerative colitis or amebiasis.

Consistency

Colonic diarrhea has foamy, floating, mucoid stools; secretory: liquid; malabsorption: soft, floating.

Color

Black or tarry stools are indicative of upper gastrointestinal bleeding unless the patient is on oral iron preparations or bismuth drugs; pale, pasty stools indicate decreased liver/gallbladder function.

Gross blood

Indicative of bowel mucosal wall destruction as in inflammatory, in-

	fectious or neoplastic disease; not psychogenic in origin. Consider the possibility of bleeding hemorrhoids.
Oil	Indicative of maldigestion, pancreatic insufficiency.
Mucus	If nonbloody, more indicative of irritable colon; functional disease.
Pus, exudate	Suggests the cause is an inflammatory or infectious process, e.g. ulcerative colitis, amebiasis, Shigella. Viral or functional disease is unlikely.
Undigested meat fibers	Indicative of maldigestion, pancreatic insufficiency.

Time

Day only	Consider functional origin.
Nighttime	Suggests organic disease. If nighttime diarrhea is associated with fecal incontinence this suggests diabetic neuropathy.
After meals	Indicative of carbohydrate intolerance, dumping syndrome.

Course

Progressive	Indicative of inflammatory, infectious disease.
Intermittent	Suggests functional disease, diabetes, Giardia.
Resolving	Possibly self-limited disease.
Stable/unchanged	Suggests inflammatory or functional disease.

Precipitated by

Medications

May be related to 1) proliferation of resistant microorganisms, 2) lincomycin (Lincocin) or clindamycin (Cleocin) induced enterocolitis, 3) side effects without pathology as in digitalis or thyroid toxicity, 4) laxative use with resulting malabsorption.

Stress, environmental changes

Suggests functional condition; obtain a detailed psychosocial history.

Particular foods

Consider food allergies: lactose intolerance is related to ingestion of milk and heavy sugar loads and occurs most commonly in nonwhite races. Consider the possibility of staphylococcal food poisoning.

Increased activity

Is associated with rectal irritation; tenesmus.

Unusual water source

Suggests parasitic or bacterial etiology.

Relieved by

Medications
  Antibiotics

Effective in tropical sprue, blind loop syndrome.

Antidiarrheal agents

Response may be helpful in planning further therapy.

Fasting

If diarrhea persists with fasting, this implies a secretory cause; if relieved with fasting, it indicates osmotic diarrhea, e.g. malabsorption, dumping syndrome.

Decreased stress

Consider functional etiology.

Nothing	Obtain a complete history of attempted therapy to plan future therapy.

Associated with

Cramping/abdominal pain	Does not occur in sprue, laxative abuse.
Urgency, tenesmus	Suggests colonic disease with rectal involvement; not found in functional disease.
Fever, chills, sweats	Suggests systemic disease, infectious process.
Nausea, vomiting	Suggests gastroenteritis, obstruction, diabetic neuropathy.
Weakness, hot flashes	Associated with dumping syndrome, carcinoid disease.
Intermittent constipation	Suggests functional syndrome, diabetic neuropathy.
Marked weight loss	Indicative of giardiasis, malabsorption, tumor, inflammatory etiology.
Travel exposure, out of country, to mountains	This may give a clue to an infectious etiology.
Family or associates with same problem (especially after ingestion of particular meal)	Suggests 1) infectious cause such as staphylococcus, botulism, Salmonella, Shigella, amebae or 2) metallic toxins: arsenic, cadmium.

Past Medical History

	Provides an overview of patient's health status affecting present illness.
Past history of diarrhea	The treatment and course of past episodes may be helpful in determining the etiology of the present problem.

Other illnesses associated
with diarrhea

Diabetes with neuropathy	Diarrhea often intermittent, often with nocturnal fecal incontinence.
Thyrotoxicosis	May cause increased motility and rapid transit.
Hypoparathyroidism	After thyroidectomy, may have cramps, tetany and steatorrhea.
Addison's disease	Symptoms: steatorrhea, weight loss.
Scleroderma	Gastrointestinal involvement results in a malabsorption state with bacterial overgrowth.
Heart disease, atherosclerosis	Associated with ischemic bowel disease.
Arthritis	Associated with colitis, Crohn's disease.

Other gastrointestinal diseases associated with diarrhea	These conditions may be associated with:
Gallstones	Crohn's disease.
Pancreatitis	Malabsorption.
Zollinger-Ellison syndrome	Increased gastric acid, decreased pH of small intestine and thus decreased absorption.
Liver disease	Crohn's disease, cancer, ulcerative colitis.
Perianal fistula/abscess	Crohn's disease.

Past abdominal surgery	Vagotomy may be associated with steatorrhea and disturbed motility.
	Gastric resection may result in dumping syndrome.
	Small bowel resection may result in changed bacterial flora, increased transit or malabsorption.
Previous hospitalizations	May provide insight into severity of present problem and other major illnesses the patient may have had.
Medications	A knowledge of medication use is indispensable in managing any illness. Some medicine may cause diarrhea (e.g. antacids, guanethidine).

OBJECTIVE DATA:

Vital signs
  Temperature
  Pulse rate
  Respiratory rate
  Blood pressure
	Fever and elevated pulse are indicative of systemic disease, infectious or inflammatory process. Postural hypotension is associated with dehydration and diabetes. Increased respiratory rate may be seen with systemic toxicity, severe pain or metabolic acidosis.

Weight	Weight is necessary to document gains/losses and severity of illiness.

Abdominal Exam

Inspection
  Scars, looseness
  of skin folds
	Indication of past surgeries, wasting disease and dehydration.

Asymmetry	Lack of symmetry is indicative of enlarged liver, spleen or tumor.

Abnormal bulging/ distention	Bulging is indicative of enlarged organ, tumor or mass. Distention indicates ascites or increased gas.
Visible peristaltic waves	Marked increase suggests obstruction.
Auscultation	Performed prior to percussion and palpation to accurately assess bowel sounds.
Bowel sounds	Hyperactive or high-pitched bowel sounds suggest small intestine disease or partial to nearly complete obstruction. If decreased or absent, suggests complete obstruction, peritonitis or ileus. Hyperactive bowel sounds may be found in viral gastroenteritis.
Friction rub	If present over the spleen, suggests infarction; if present over the liver, suggests hepatoma or metastatic cancer.
Bruits	These may suggest arterial narrowing with vascular insufficiency, arteriovenous malformation or a large tumor.
Palpation Mass	Consider tumor, stool in bowel or impaction; if tenderness is present consider diverticulitis with complicating abscess.
Liver palpable	Suggests cirrhosis, hepatitis or tumor.
Spleen palpable	Consider hepatitis, portal hypertension.

Tenderness, rebound	Rebound tenderness is indicative of peritonitis. Right lower quadrant local, tender mass suggests regional enteritis (terminal ileum) or appendicitis.
	Liver tenderness suggests amebiasis or hepatitis. Local tender mass suggests inflamed diverticulum.
Rigidity	Indicative of intestinal perforation, peritonitis, "surgical abdomen."
Fluid wave	Indicative of free fluid in abdomen (ascites).
Percussion	
Percussed resonance	There is normal increased tympany over hollow organs, the stomach, or with increased gas and distended bowel. Increased dullness occurs over tumor or solid organs.
Shifting dullness	Characteristic of ascites.

Rectal Examination

External hemorrhoids	Observe for source of gross blood.
Fistula/abscess	Associated with inflammatory bowel disease.
Sphincter tone	If decreased, may be associated with neuropathy.
Tenderness	If present, indicative of an inflammatory process in large bowel diarrhea. Most prominent with ulcerative colitis, gonorrheal proctitis, perirectal abscess. Not present in functional disease.

Impaction	If present, may be mechanical basis for diarrhea.

General Examination

Inappropriate affect	Observe for clues to emotional problems.
Dehydration signs	Helpful to determine severity of diarrhea and need for fluid therapy and electrolyte replacement.
Increased skin pigmentation	Associated with sprue, Addison's disease.
Weight loss evidence (wasting, poor skin turgor)	Associated with severe acute diarrhea, tumor, ulcerative colitis, giardiasis or malabsorption.
Thyroid disease	Diarrhea may be associated with hyperthyroidism.
Lymphadenopathy	Associated with systemic disease, lymphoma.
Neurologic examination	Diabetes and amyloidosis may be associated with diarrhea. Neurological exam reveals signs of peripheral neuropathy, especially in the legs.

Lab Data
Gross Stool Examination

Blood	Indicative of hemorrhoids, tumor, diverticula, inflammatory or infectious disease; not present in functional disease.
Pus	Indicative of infectious process and/or some inflammatory diseases.
Mucus	Indicative of ulcerative colitis, irritable bowel.

Oil, meat fibers	Occurs with maldigestion, pancreatic insufficiency.
Hematest	Occult blood indicates gastrointestinal bleeding.

Microscopic Stool Examination

Ova, parasite	Indicates specific infectious etiology.
RBC's, WBC's	Indicative of infectious and/or inflammatory etiology, particularly if polymorphonuclear cells predominate.
Odor	If odorous, suggests fat malabsorption.
Sudan stain	Indicates the presence of oils, thus implying malabsorption of fat.

Other Lab

CBC with Differential	To evaluate for systemic disease, associated anemia or infectious etiology (increased WBC).
Electrolytes/BUN	To evaluate hydration and electrolyte status. Abnormalities suggest severe diarrhea. Significant diarrhea may decrease serum potassium.
Urinalysis	Specific gravity is increased with dehydration if renal function is normal. Glycosuria indicates diabetes. Presence of bilirubin indicates liver disease.

Radiology

3 way of abdomen	Observe for: 1) air-fluid levels indicative of paralytic ileus, obstruction; 2) pancreatic calcification indicative of chronic pan-

creatitis; 3) calcified lymph nodes suggestive of tuberculosis, histoplasmosis; 4) air under diaphragm indicative of perforation.

ASSESSMENT:

The etiology of diarrhea can be classified into several broad groups, although these categories are not necessarily mutually exclusive. Only the common, frequently seen causes will be reviewed in detail.

Acute Diarrhea

Characterized by sudden, often explosive onset, with symptoms lasting a few hours to several days. If diarrhea persists longer than 5-7 days, a more extensive evaluation is needed. Additional diagnostic data include stool for ova and parasite, and culture and sensitivity.

Toxic diarrhea

Characterized by abrupt onset, generalized abdominal cramps, often associated with nausea, vomiting, explosive stools which are usually large volume and nonbloody. There may be a history of close associates with similar symptoms after a common meal. *Etiology:* staphylococcus, enteropathogenic *E. coli,* cholera, *Clostridium perfringens* or chemical poisons such as arsenic, lead, mercury, cadmium.

Infectious diarrhea
Salmonella

8-48 hours after ingestion of contaminated food there is the onset of fever, nausea, vomiting, abdominal pain and diarrhea. Stools are often slimy, with a green pea soup appearance. At onset, stools rarely

	have blood or mucus. This is a self-limiting illness. Host: livestock, poultry, man.
Shigella	Usually self-limiting. Characterized by abdominal pain, fever and bloody mucoid stools 1-3 days after onset. Host: contaminated food or water; man.
Enteropathogenic *E. coli*	Occurs most commonly in children but recent evidence indicates adult disease is common. May be the major cause of travelers' diarrhea.
Abnormal bowel flora	Usually occurs after antibiotic therapy due to proliferation of resistant strains of staphylococcus, Proteus, Pseudomonas, streptococcus or fungus growth such as Candida.
Virus	Acute onset, duration 2-3 days, no exudate with stools. Viral culture is specific for diagnosis. Associated with systemic symptoms.
Parasites *Giardia lamblia*	Infests small intestine, interferes with fat absorption. Symptoms may be intermittent. Stool may contain fat and mucus. Acute onset, can become chronic with noticable weight loss.
Amebiasis	Caused by *E. histolytica,* characterized by ulcers of colon, severe, bloody, mucoid stools, low grade fever, abdominal pain. May be precipitated by stress, climate or diet changes. Carrier state is often asymptomatic. A large, tender liver may indicate abscess.

Acute episodes of chronic diarrhea	See Chronic Diarrhea for descriptions.
Dietary	Caused by: a. Irritating or allergenic foods: lactose or disaccharide intolerance. b. Drug: antibiotics, antacids, opiate withdrawal, cathartics, antimetabolites, cholinergics.
Other causes	Acute gastrointestinal bleed, mesenteric infarction, appendicitis, pericolonic or perirectal abscess.
Chronic Diarrhea	Often characterized by insidious onset, although may be sudden; persisting for months to years.
Small bowel	Generally characterized by 1-4 stools daily, nonviolent, lacking urgency, tenesmus, mucus or nocturnal stools. If abdominal cramps present, they are mild to moderate and periumbilical; steatorrhea is often present. Diagnostic tests are directed to suspected cause.
Malabsorption	The small intestine functions abnormally and passes a large bulk to the colon. The colon is unable to reabsorb the increased amount of fluid and electrolytes. Specifically, the colon cannot reabsorb: a. Fats in pancreatic insufficiency, sprue, celiac disease. The resulting stool is bulky, pale and greasy, has increased odor, and is floating or foaming. b. Carbohydrates resulting in an osmotic diarrhea. Lactose is not broken down with resulting watery stools from increased osmot-

117

ic pressure in the small intestine. The same process occurs with certain laxatives. This disorder is a result of decreased mucosal lactase activity. It is most common in nonwhite races. The patient often gives a personal or family history of milk intolerance.

Secretory

Due to increased liquid stool volume secreted into the small intestine which is unable to reabsorb it.

a. Zollinger-Ellison syndrome (gastric ulcer syndrome). Diarrhea occurs as a result of increased gastric acidity (decreased pH) with resulting decreased fat digestion and osmotic diarrhea.

b. Pancreatic tumor. Diarrhea is the result of hormone secretion of pancreatic islet cell tumors causing marked watery diarrhea up to 6 liters a day. With acute episodes, dehydration and hypokalemia are common. The hormone affects intestinal water and electrolyte transport and inhibits gastric acid secretion, with resulting high levels of potassium and low levels of sodium in the stool.

Motility disorder

a. Hyperthyroidism has associated diarrhea. This is probably caused by increased smooth muscle activity, with resulting increased gastric emptying and increased intestinal motility, causing decreased transit time and some malabsorption.

b. Carcinoid syndrome occurs with diarrhea as the prominent symptom. This is a result of tumor secretion of serotonin causing intestinal hypertrophy.

c. Dumping syndrome. Associated diarrhea results from a hyperosmotic solution introduced into the proximal jejunum causing increased small intestine secretions and increased peristalsis. The watery stools characteristically occur soon after meals.

Colonic diarrhea

Characterized by 3-12 stools daily or passage of blood and/or mucus, with marked urgency and tenesmus and lower abdominal cramps which are relieved by bowel movement. Occurs frequently after meals or may occur at night. If rectal inflammation is present, there may be fecal incontinence. Additional diagnostic tools include stool examination for ova and parasites, culture and sensitivity; sigmoidoscopy and barium enema.

Inflammatory disease

a. *Infectious:* Salmonella, Shigella, *E. Histolytica* as described under acute syndrome.

b. *Ulcerative colitis:* Frequent bloody mucoid stools, ulcers in colonic mucosa, malaise, anorexia, weight loss and perhaps fever. With ulcers, hemorrhage or perforation may occur. Exacerbation occurs with stress and/or diet change.

c. *Regional enteritis (Crohn's disease):* Involves any area of the intestine; may be ulcerative. Acute symptoms include frequent, watery, light-colored stools, abdominal pain and increased flatus. Chronicity may lead to partial bowel obstruction, local abscess and fistula formation from bowel to abdominal wall or other loops of bowel or anal skin. May have a right lower quadrant tender mass related to the inflammatory process.

d. *Diverticulitis:* Inflammation of an outpouching sac in the colon wall. There is left sided abdominal pain and tenderness; pericolonic abscess may develop with inflammation of the peritoneum; or perforation with resulting picture of "acute abdomen" can occur.

Neurogenic diarrhea

Caused by autonomic nerve degeneration. Intermittent symptoms make this condition difficult to diagnose and treat.

Diabetic neuropathy

Occurs in patients with peripheral neuropathy, i.e. with diabetes which has been difficult to control for more than 5 years. Stools are watery; often nocturnal with fecal incontinence; with or without steatorrhea; occasionally bloody. Alternates with constipation. Diabetic neuropathy is associated with impotence, postural hypotension, bladder dysfunction. The etiology is unknown, possibly related to poor carbohydrate absorption, increased bacterial flora and/or altered motility.

Amyloidosis

Associated with peripheral neuropathy or autonomic dysfunction in the nondiabetic. Has widespread intestinal infiltration and may involve destruction of the pancreas. Symptoms are similar to diabetic neuropathy.

Functional diarrhea

Characterized by intermittent constipation and diarrhea, which is a life-long pattern. Stools are small volume, often small and pellet-like (from spasm), nonbloody, foul smelling and not nocturnal. Often accompanied by distention, bloating, increased flatus and inconsistent food intolerance. Associated with anxiety, depression and stress. There is no marked weight loss and gastrointestinal work-up is negative. Most commonly occurs in young women.

Other causes

1. Impinging colonic tumor causing obstruction.
2. Bowel as the primary site of scleroderma.
3. Endocrine:
    Addison's disease
    Hypoparathyroidism
    Thyrotoxicosis
4. Blind loop syndrome: bacterial overgrowth in a stagnant loop of bowel leads to malabsorption. Associated with diabetes, scleroderma, gastrointestinal surgery and small bowel diverticula.

PLAN:

Diagnostic
    Stool ova and parasites
        Culture and sensitivity

To rule out infectious process. Consider doing if history of symptoms is more than 48 hours.

72 hour stool for fat	To document malabsorption.
Blood studies CBC with differential	WBC is elevated with inflammatory or infectious process. Also done to rule out associated anemia.
Electrolytes/BUN	To evaluate dehydration, acidosis and potassium level.
Glucose	To rule out diabetic etiology.
Thyroid function tests	To rule out thyroid disease.

Sigmoidoscopy

1. Indicated in prolonged diarrhea of unknown etiology or in grossly bloody or purulent diarrhea.
2. To rule out mucosal inflammation, ulcers, tumor, polyps; not helpful with malabsorption syndrome.
3. To obtain mucosal smears for pus of inflammatory disease.
4. To obtain biopsy as needed.

Radiology
  Barium enema

Helps define lesions and extent of colon disease (ulcerative colitis, diverticula). To rule out tumors; to visualize terminal ileum for diagnosis of regional enteritis.

Upper gastrointestinal series with small bowel follow through

Usually abnormal with malabsorption, regional enteritis.

Therapeutic
  Criteria for
  hospitalization

1. Significant dehydration when diarrhea is not resolving.
2. Signs of marked toxicity, e.g. high fever, elevated WBC.

3. New diagnosis or exacerbation of ulcerative colitis or regional enteritis.

Treatment plan

1. Bedrest to decrease peristalsis.
2. *Diet:* Low fat, low residue; increased fluids to achieve bowel rest. With upper bowel symptoms, avoiding cold fluids may decrease bowel motility.
3. *Remove causative factors,* e.g. food, stress, medications. This is particularly helpful in chronic diarrhea.
4. *Drugs:*
   a. *Kaolin-pectin (Kaopectate):* Acts as an absorbent to bind gas and bacteria.
   b. Anticholinergics such as belladonna are effective in decreasing motility of functional bowel syndrome; they are ineffective with infectious or inflammatory disease.
   c. *Diphenoxylate (Lomotil):* Acts by working on gastrointestinal smooth muscle, thus decreasing bowel motility. It may be contraindicated if the etiologic agent is invasive to bowel lining; e.g. Shigella. With invasive bowel disease, Lomotil can prolong the carrier state of the disease and lengthen the clinical course of symptoms by decreasing motility, thus allowing increased penetration of bacteria into the mucosal wall. In ulcerative colitis, Lomotil may precipitate toxic megacolon.

d. *Opiates:* Act to decrease bowel motility. Serve as bowel analgesic. Same contraindications as Lomotil.

e. *Antibiotics:* Used in some severe infectious or inflammatory processes although use is not well defined. May be indicated in debilitated patients. In severe Shigella and Salmonella infections, especially typhoid, antiobiotics may be useful, but may lengthen carrier state.

f. Other drugs are very specific for specific diarrheal diseases: Flagyl for Giardia infection, steroids for severe ulcerative colitis and regional enteritis. Antiemetics may be used for nausea and vomiting associated with diarrhea.

g. IV fluids may be necessary with severe dehydration.

Patient education

Return if the diarrhea worsens, bloody stools develop, fever/shaking chills occur, if unable to retain fluids (dehydration) or if diarrhea persists more than 5-7 days. Occurrence of above may require examination by a gastroenterologist or hospitalization.

Call for test results, especially stool O & P, C & S in 2 days or when available.

If contagious, instruct regarding stool precautions.

Explain necessity of returning for reculture until clear of infectious cause.

Explain need for referral to a gastroenterologist for diagnosis and specific treatment if indicated.

BIBLIOGRAPHY

Dupont, Herbert L., and Richard B. Hornick: "Clinical Approach to Infectious Diarrheas," *Medicine,* 52:4, pp. 265-270, 1973.

Dupont, Herbert L., and Richard B. Hornick: "Diarrheal Diseases," *Disease-a-Month,* pp. 3-40, July 1969.

Harrison, T. R. (ed.): "Constipation and Diarrhea," *Principles of Internal Medicine,* 7th ed., New York, McGraw-Hill, 1974.

Katz, Leonard A., and Howard A. Spiro: "Medical Progress: GI Manifestations of Diabetes," *New England Journal of Medicine,* 275:24, pp. 1350-1361, 1966.

MacBryde, C. M. (ed.): "Constipation and Diarrhea," *Signs and Symptoms,* 5th ed., Philadelphia, Lippincott, pp. 381-397, 1970.

Phillips, S. F.: "Diarrhea: A Current View of Pathophysiology," *Gastroenterology,* 63: pp. 495-511, September 1972.

Sleisenger, Marvin H., and John S. Fordtran: *Gastrointestinal Disease,* Philadelphia, Saunders, pp. 308-317, 1973.

NOTES

Dizziness/
vertigo

DIZZINESS/VERTIGO WORKSHEET

To be used for patients with:
Wooziness/Giddiness
Lightheadedness
Fainting
Sensation of Spinning
Sensation of Swimming

What you can't afford to miss: CNS lesion, acute otitis media, significant arrhythmia.

Chief Complaint: _____

SUBJECTIVE DATA:

Character, describe: _____Vertigo: _____Yes _____No

Onset: _____Sudden _____Gradual _____Date of onset

Duration: _____Constant _____Episodic

_____Duration of each episode

Frequency (number of episodes): _____

Relieved by: _____

DESCRIBE POSITIVE RESPONSES
(Include Onset, Severity, Duration)

PRECIPITATED BY:
Yes   No

___ ___ Position (head or body movement): _____

___ ___ Meals: _____

___ ___ Trauma: _____Head/neck _____When

___ ___ Physical exertion:_____

___ ___ Emotional stress/anxiety: _____

___ ___ Rapid breathing (hyperventilation): _____

___ ___ Other: _____

ASSOCIATED WITH:
Yes   No

___ ___ Noises in ear (tinnitus):_____

___ ___ Hearing loss: _____

___ ___ Ear discharge: _____

___ ___ Fullness in ear:_____

___ ___ Headache: _____

___ ___ Photophobia: _____

___ ___ Diplopia:_____

___ ___ Scotomata: _____

___ ___ Blurred vision: _____

___ ___ Dental problems:_____

Protocols for Common Acute Self-Limiting Problems

___ ___ Nausea/vomiting: _____

___ ___ Menstrual irregularities: _____

___ ___ Loss of balance/difficulty walking: _____

___ ___ Fainting: _____

___ ___ Disturbance in coordination: _____

___ ___ Paralysis: _____

___ ___ Generalized weakness: _____

___ ___ Flu/cold/sinusitis: _____

___ ___ Fever: _____

___ ___ Increased number of infections: _____

___ ___ Polyphagia, polydipsia, polyuria: _____

___ ___ Nervousness: _____

___ ___ Heart trouble, palpitations, skipping: _____

___ ___ Hypertension: _____

PAST MEDICAL HISTORY:
Yes *No*

___ ___ Cardiovascular problems: _____

___ ___ Neurological problems: _____

___ ___ Endocrine problems: _____

___ ___ Hematopoietic problems: _____

___ ___ Use of medications: _____

___ ___ Allergies: _____

FAMILY HISTORY:
Yes   *No*

___   ___   Cardiovascular problems: _____

___   ___   Central nervous system disorders: _____

___   ___   Endocrine problems: _____

___   ___   Headaches: _____

SOCIAL HISTORY:
Yes   *No*

___   ___   Smoking: _____

___   ___   Alcohol: _____

___   ___   Caffeine: _____

___   ___   Stressful situations: _____

___   ___   Travel (airplane, mountains): _____

OBJECTIVE DATA:
Vital Signs: ___B/P Lying ___Standing (immediately)

         ___Standing (3 minutes) ___P ___R ___T ___Wt

General appearance (signs of anxiousness, nervousness, hyper-

activity): _____

_____

_____

DESCRIBE POSITIVE RESPONSES

EAR EXAM: _____Not Done
Yes   *No*

___   ___   Hearing deficit: _____Weber _____Rinne

____ ____ Occlusion of external canals: _____

____ ____ Tympanic membrane (perforated, retracted, bulging):

_____

NOSE, MOUTH, THROAT, NECK EXAM: _____Not Done
Yes　*No*

____ ____ Nasal discharge: _____

____ ____ Sinus tenderness:_____

____ ____ Sinus transillumination abnormal:_____

____ ____ Malocclusion of bite: _____

____ ____ Temporomandibular joint tenderness:_____

____ ____ Poor dental repair: _____

____ ____ Pharynx red; exudate:_____

____ ____ Tonsils (tonsillar pillars) edematous; exudate:_____

_____

____ ____ Neck adenopathy: _____

____ ____ Cervical vertebral or muscle tenderness: _____

____ ____ Decreased range of motion in neck:_____

EYE EXAM: _____Not Done
Yes　*No*

____ ____ Decreased visual acuity: _____

____ ____ Decreased visual fields:_____

____ ____ Presence of cataracts: _____

____ ____ Abnormalities of fundus: _____

____ ____ Extraocular movement deficit: _____

____ ____ Nystagmus (with extraocular movements or postural tests):

_____

NEUROLOGICAL EXAM: _____Not Done

Yes   No

____ ____ Cerebral function deficit (mental status)

(specify how tested): _____

____ ____ Cranial nerve deficit (specify results of exam):

_____I _____II _____III, IV, VI

_____V _____VII _____VIII _____IX

_____X _____XI _____XII

____ ____ Decreased motor function, range of motion:

_____

____ ____ Sensory deficits: _____

____ ____ Cerebellar dysfunction:
past pointing, fine coordination (finger to nose, RAM),
balance (Romberg)

Describe gait: _____

_____

____ ____ Reflexes (hypo/hyperactivity, absence): _____

_____

CARDIOVASCULAR EXAM: _____Not Done

Yes   *No*

____   ____   Arrhythmias: _____

____   ____   Carotid pulse deficit: _____

____   ____   Great vessel bruits: _____

____   ____   Varicose veins: _____

____   ____   Edema:_____

DIZZINESS SIMULATION TESTS: _____Not Done
  (dizziness can be simulated with following tests)

Yes   *No*

____   ____   Change in posture: _____

____   ____   Carotid sinus stimulation:_____

____   ____   Turning head: _____

____   ____   Hyperventilation:_____

____   ____   Valsalva maneuver: _____

____   ____   Sudden turn when walking:_____

____   ____   Sitting/standing with eyes open and closed:_____

    _____

____   ____   Positional vertigo maneuver: _____

LAB DATA:
Done   *Not*
     Done

____   ____   Urinalysis: _____

____   ____   CBC:_____

___ ___ Blood sugar: _____

___ ___ Electrolytes: _____

___ ___ X-Rays: _____Cervical spine

_____Skull

___ ___ Electrocardiogram: _____

___ ___ Other: _____

ASSESSMENT:

_____

_____

_____

_____

PLAN:
DIAGNOSTIC:

_____T_3/T_4

_____Lumbar puncture

_____ENT consult

_____Neurologic consult

_____Orthopedic consult

_____Cardiovascular consult

_____Psychiatric consult

THERAPEUTIC:

_____

_____

_____

_____

PATIENT EDUCATION:

_____Identification of stresses: _____

_____Explain test results:_____

_____Explain treatment: _____

_____Other: _____

DIZZINESS/VERTIGO WORKSHEET RATIONALE

Complaints of dizziness can be categorized in four ways:

1. *Vertigo:* The person experiences a sensation of rotation; or his environment, though stationary, appears to move.
2. *Syncope:* A sensation of impending faintness or loss of consciousness.
3. *Disequilibrium:* A sensation of loss of balance (no head involvement).
4. *Dizziness:* An unpleasant sensation of disturbed relationship to surrounding objects. This may be an ill-defined feeling of light-headedness, giddiness, a swimming sensation, mental confusion or wooziness.

The terms vertigo and dizziness are often used interchangeably and both are expressions of a balance disturbance. The system responsible for maintaining balance is composed of three body senses: vision, muscle and joint proprioceptors and the vestibular system. These sensory systems interact to adjust and counteract the opposing forces of motion and gravity. The central nervous system is involved in the integration of responses from these three senses.

The end organs of the vestibular system, housed in the inner ear, are collectively called the labyrinth and are most often the origin of balance disturbance. However, because of the series of connections from the labyrinth, such as to the eyes, the deep and superficial positional receptors, the spine, the cortex, the cerebellum, the autonomic nervous system and reticular formation, there are many other pathologic possibilities for the cause of dizziness.

The etiological basis of dizziness can be neurologic, cardiac, hematologic, vascular, psychiatric or ophthalmologic, as well as due to peripheral vestibular disorders. One study[1] of 108 patients presenting with the complaint of dizziness showed the following breakdown of etiologies:

Peripheral vestibular disorders	38 %
Hyperventilation syndrome	23 %
Multiple sensory deficits	13 %
Psychogenic dizziness	9 %
Uncertain diagnosis	9 %
Brainstem cerebrovascular accident	5 %
Cardiovascular	4 %
Other neurologic disorders	4 %
Multiple sclerosis	2 %
Visual problems	2 %
Endocrine problems	1 %
Excessive awareness of normal sensation	1 %

Some patients had more than one diagnosis, thus the percentages add up to more than 100 per cent.

Dizziness originating in the peripheral apparatus occurs more frequently than does that of central origin. However, causes originating in the labyrinth are not life-threatening, whereas dizziness originating in the central nervous system may be serious to both health and life itself. It is important, therefore, to first evaluate the possibility of central nervous system disorders when examining a patient with dizziness.

SUBJECTIVE DATA:

Character

Dizziness is a vague term used to describe many sensations. It is necessary to determine whether true vertigo (motion sensation) is

[1]Drachman, David A., and Cecil W. Hart, "An Approach to the Dizzy Patient," *Neurology*, Vol. 22, No. 4, April, 1972, pp. 323-334.

present. Generally, vertigo is present with 8th cranial nerve involvement (peripheral disease) and not with central nervous system disease. The closer the lesion is to the peripheral labyrinth, the more active the vertigo. It is thought by some that the direction of the rotation of vertigo in a peripheral disease is toward the unaffected side; the direction of the rotation of vertigo in a central lesion is toward the side of the lesion.

Onset

Sudden onset vs. chronic presence gives an important clue as to origin of the symptom. A sudden primary attack in a person below age 40 is commonly caused by nonspecific labyrinthitis. In patients over 40, sudden dizziness/vertigo commonly is caused by a vascular disorder involving vertebral or basilar arteries or the internal acoustic branch of the 8th cranial nerve. The 8th cranial nerve and vestibular nuclei receive their main blood supply from basilar arteries. Consider also that a sudden attack of vertigo may follow extreme physical or emotional stress.

Duration
Number of episodes

Central nervous system disorders generally give rise to constant vertigo/dizziness, whereas labyrinthine lesions usually cause episodic attacks. With intracranial tumors, symptoms are usually constant, not intermittent. With positional vertigo, attacks last only 5-10 seconds. Episodes due to Meniere's disease last 30 minutes to hours (not days);

they are recurrent with periods of freedom from attacks for months or even years. See section on Tinnitus, p. 142.

Relieved by

With benign positional vertigo, change of position will relieve the dizziness. With cardiovascular origin, lying down will generally relieve the dizziness. In multiple sensory deficits, a stabilizing factor may be for the patient to touch another person or object.

Precipitated by
  Position (head or body
  movement)

Both peripheral and central vertigo may be influenced by position. Benign positional vertigo is the classification used when the symptom is present with specific positions, i.e. head hanging down or turned to one side or immediately upon standing. Benign positional vertigo is vestibular in origin and is diagnosed when no other definite underlying condition is present.

In the elderly, dizziness often occurs with arising in the morning. The cause is vascular and related to inability of the general circulation to adapt promptly to change in position, resulting in hypotension and decreased cerebral circulation.

Osteophytes of the cervical spine may cause dizziness upon head movement. This is due to pressure on nerves or vessels in the area.

Atherosclerotic individuals with disease affecting the head and neck vessels may suffer dizziness produced by neck turning. The cause may be narrowing of the lumen of the contralateral vertebral artery.

Meals

If dizziness occurs during a meal, consider dental malocclusions; this relates to close proximity of the acoustic nerve to the temporomandibular joint. Food allergies and dumping syndrome also can present as dizziness.

Trauma
Head/neck/spine

With trauma to the head or neck (cervical spine) the nerve tracts to the vestibular apparatus could be disturbed. Dizziness, not true vertigo, is a common complaint after head injury; the complaint usually is a feeling of unsteadiness or disturbance in equilibrium. Dizziness following trauma may be due to traumatic lesions affecting the vestibular structures in the brain stem or trauma to the inner ear apparatus. Postural vertigo may be present after whiplash, probably due to vestibular end-organ damage. If there is hemorrhage following head trauma, dizziness may be provoked by movement and accompanied by headache and vomiting.

Trauma to any part of the spinal column can produce positional imbalance identified as dizziness.

Psychological aspects associated with any head/neck trauma are also important to consider. Psychogenic factors arising out of circumstances associated with the injury may precipitate symptoms such as dizziness. Both the physical effect of the injury on structures inside the skull and the psychogenic factors associated with the injury must be considered.

Physical exertion

Cause is unknown, but empirically, physical exertion may cause dizziness.

Emotional stress/anxiety

Patients with dizziness, with a psychological disorder as the primary cause, usually give a history of constant, vague lightheadedness that may be longstanding. They will also give a history of difficulty with concentration and loss of energy, interest and appetite, and complain of fatigue. All these are signs of depression and anxiety. It is important to rule out organic disease before deciding that the origin of dizziness is psychogenic. Also consider that a person who has dizziness of unknown origin may become anxious and depressed.

Hyperventilation

Hyperventilation is a fairly common cause for dizziness. If dizziness is precipitated by hyperventilation associated with anxiety or other emotional stress, a psychosomatic diagnosis can be made after other serious disorders are ruled out. Dizziness produced by hyperventilation is not understood; possible causes are cerebral anoxia due to decreased cerebral blood flow and increased cerebral cortical irritability due to overbreathing. The hyperventilation can also be secondary to a compensatory mechanism in severe metabolic acidosis, especially diabetic ketoacidosis.

Associated with
  Tinnitus
    Hearing loss/
    ear fullness/
    ear discharge

If vertigo is constant in the presence of ear symptoms, consider acoustic neuroma and other cerebellopontine angle tumors resulting in involvement of the vestibular nerve and nuclei in the adjacent brainstem. However, with 8th nerve damage, vertigo is not a common first sign; it is usually a late manifestation accompanied by other neurological signs.

Patients with episodic, recurrent vertigo accompanied by tinnitus and hearing loss may have Meniere's disease. The underlying cause of Meniere's disease is not known, but may be due to overproduction and/or diminished resorption of endolymph. The increased endolymphatic pressure results in asphyxia of vestibular endorgans. The tinnitus is usually confined to the involved ear and worsens during an attack. Deafness is usually unilateral and of sensorineural or inner ear type; it fluctuates and decreases during an attack.

Any unilateral obstruction of the eustachian tubes may result in dizziness. The cause in this case is not exactly known, but the obstruction results in an alteration of pressure relationships that exist in the middle ears. Focal infections of the nose/throat may result in ear symptoms and can be related to the dizziness. These infections may result in blockage of the eustachian tubes. Middle ear infections may produce dizziness due to resulting imbalance between the two labyrinths. Viral labyrinthitis, an acute but benign disease, may result in dizziness accompanied by fullness in the ear, but not usually by deafness, and rarely by tinnitus.

Aspirin can cause tinnitus and dizziness.

Seasickness, once commonly thought to be ocular in origin, is now thought to be due to excessive stimulation of the inner ear.

Headache

Vertigo may present as an aura for migraine headaches. Abrupt alterations in the caliber of cerebral and meningeal arteries may cause disturbances in vestibular function. Labyrinthitis may be caused by viral or bacterial meningitis and may be associated with severe, persistent headaches as well as with dizziness.

Ocular problems
  Photophobia
  Double/blurred vision
  Decreased visual acuity

Although ocular problems are not a common primary cause of dizziness, a deficit in balance sensation may be caused by a visual defect, just as a sensory deficit can cause loss of perspective to environment. Visual defects may cause a discrepancy between visual perception and proprioceptive impulses. Thus, for some people, being at heights or watching moving objects may bring on dizziness.

Blurred vision is commonly found with vertigo. If diplopia is present, it indicates other visual or oculomotor system disturbance.

Dental problems

The cause of dizziness may be dental malocclusal and temporomandibular joint abnormalities due to close proximity of anatomical structures to vestibular conductive systems and auditory systems. An abscessed tooth may be the source of an infectious process involving the vestibule.

Nausea/vomiting

With a labyrinth disorder, vertigo is frequently associated with nausea and vomiting. If nausea and vomiting is present without pain or hearing loss and with no neurological dysfunction, consider occlusion of labyrinth division of the internal auditory artery. Vertigo with origin in the brainstem is associated with headaches and vomiting which precede the onset of vertigo.

Menstrual irregularities

Vasomotor reactions occurring during the menopause may be associated with dizziness. Anemia resulting from menorrhagia may produce dizziness on an anoxic basis.

Loss of balance, coordination; unsteady gait

If continuous ataxia is present between dizzy spells, origin of dizziness is probably not a labyrinthine lesion, and neurological conditions are suspected. Persons with a tumor of the 8th cranial nerve may describe dizziness as an unsteady feeling rather than true vertigo. In lesions of the cerebellum, the vestibular connection in the posterior vermis may be involved, with resulting disturbances of equilibrium and coordination. People with supratentorial vascular accidents, with consciousness retained, may complain of lightheadedness or an unsteady sensation rather than true vertigo.

Cardiovascular disorders and blood diseases may produce a feeling of unsteadiness, swimming or lightheadedness; most often these sensations are relieved by lying down. The cause may be imperfect vasomotor adjustment of diseased blood vessels or cerebral anoxia secondary to transitory ischemia. Anoxia from circulatory disorders in the vestibular pathway can produce dizziness. Stenosis of vertebral and basilar arteries resulting in ischemia of the brainstem may produce ataxia and leg weakness, among other neurological signs.

Orthopedic disorders need to be considered with ambulation problems.

Patients with multiple sensory deficits may become confused when walking, lose balance or position perspective and experience dizziness. Multiple sensory deficits are defined as two or more of the following:
1. Neuropathy (especially diabetic).

2. Noncorrectable visual impairment.
3. Vestibular deficits.
4. Cervical spondylosis (symptoms on turning head).
5. Orthopedic disorders interfering with ambulation.

Damage to the spinal column following trauma may produce dizziness or balance loss.

Fainting

Syncope does not occur with labyrinthine disease. With syncope in the presence of persistent vertigo, headaches and obscured vision, consider vertebral-basilar artery insufficiency. If the patient has a history of cardiac problems and presents with vertigo and syncope, suspect cardiac arrhythmias which result in inadequate cerebral blood supply.

Patients with carotid sinus hypersensitivity may experience syncope associated with vertigo when holding the neck to one side or the other.

Occasionally, epileptic attacks may be preceded by vertigo or dizziness; the vertigo or dizziness represents an aura to seizures.

Paralysis/tingling

Suspect underlying neurological disease. Facial paralysis with dizziness may occur in multiple sclerosis involving the brainstem. With cerebrovascular stenosis of vertebral and basilar arteries, tingling of the face may occur. With hyperventilation, perioral and finger paresthesias may occur.

Generalized weakness/ fever	Generalized weakness and fever are often nonspecific complaints of systemic disease, e.g. infections. Weakness associated with dizziness may also be a sign of hypoglycemia.
	Hematopoietic conditions resulting in decreased oxygen delivery to the brain may present with vague symptoms of weakness, headache and dizziness.
Flu/cold/sinusitis	Infectious processes, especially of the upper respiratory tract, may disturb function of the vestibular apparatus and cause dizziness.
Polyphagia/ polydipsia/polyuria	Patients with previously undiagnosed diabetes mellitus often present with vague symptoms of dizziness.
Nervousness/anxiousness	In addition to emotional stress, these symptoms could indicate thyroid problems such as myxedema, which causes endolymph fluid changes in the inner ear and produces dizziness.
Cardiovascular problems Palpitations Skipping beats Shortness of breath	Impaired circulation resulting in cerebral anoxia is the general cause of dizziness with cardiovascular problems.
Hypertension	Drugs used for cardiovascular diseases, particularly for hypertension, are often the cause of dizziness. With hypertension, the exact cause of dizziness is unknown but may be sudden marked fluctuations in blood pressure causing recurrent local circulatory insufficiency in the

vestibular system. Another theory holds that vasospasm associated with hypertensive vascular disease may result in dizziness.

Also see Fainting, Loss of balance and Position.

Past Medical History

As indicated in previous discussion, any past history in these specific areas may give a clue to the cause of dizziness:

Cardiovascular: arteriosclerotic disease, hypertension.

Neurological: epilepsy, strokes, sensory deficits.

Endocrine: diabetes, thyroid disorders.

Hematopoietic: anemia, blood dyscrasias.

Orthopedic problems: interference with ambulation.

Ear problems, eye problems: see previous discussion for details.

Migraine headaches: dizziness may be aura for headaches.

Psychological problems: see previous discussion for details.

Essentially, the total body may be under suspicion!

Medications

Streptomycin directly damages the 8th cranial nerve. Drug poisoning, especially by salicylates, may cause dizziness through effects on the central nervous system center which produces hyperventilation, resulting in respiratory alkalosis and dizziness. Other drugs may also produce dizziness, particularly antihypertensives, hormones, sedatives, tranquilizers, diuretics, antihistamines and nasal sprays.

Allergies

Information about allergies influences the treatment plan. Also, history of allergies to drugs or other antigens may show causal relationship to the dizziness.

Family History

Many of the conditions discussed above, specifically arteriosclerotic heart disease, epilepsy, diabetes, migraine headaches, have familial tendencies and may be clues to the patient's underlying condition.

Social History
Smoking
Alcohol
Caffeine

Constriction or dilatation of blood vessels produced by these agents may cause dizziness. Smoking also increases carbon monoxide levels, which may produce dizziness. Information about cigarette use can also be important in determining the patient's risk for developing cardiovascular and cerebrovascular problems, as smoking is a precursor for these diseases.

Stressful situations

It may be necessary to elicit a thorough life-style social history to detect stressful situations associated with the dizziness; the patient often is not aware of stress he is experiencing.

Travel by air or in mountains	Alterations of pressure in the middle ear may be the origin of dizziness.

OBJECTIVE DATA:

Vital signs

Specifically, look for hypertension, postural hypotension, arrhythmias, fever or any other indication of cardiovascular problem or infectious process.

General appearance

Look for signs of anxiousness, nervousness or hyperactivity. Also, evaluate whether the dizziness or vertigo is incapacitating.

Ear Exam
Hearing deficit
Weber/Rinne

See subjective information for rationale in relation to vertigo/dizziness with ear problems. Any ear problem may have a direct relationship to dizziness.

Hearing loss may be due to conductive loss through impaction or other obstruction, or a sensorineural loss.

Hearing perception and conduction are tested with the Weber and Rinne tests.

Weber: Lateralization of sound to one ear indicates conductive loss in that ear or neural loss in the other ear.

Rinne: Air conduction should be twice as long as bone conduction in each ear. Abnormalities in this test are:

1. Poor bone conduction, which will make air conduction longer than twice that of bone conduction.

2. Obstruction of the canal or middle ear making air conduction shorter than bone conduction.

External canals
Tympanic membranes

Look for signs of occlusion, inflammation and perforation.

Nose/mouth/throat/neck

Look for signs of upper respiratory infection or localized problem such as abscess or trauma in these areas. Because of close proximity to vestibular apparatus of the ear these may be related to dizziness or vertigo. See Subjective Rationale for flu/cold/sinusitis, trauma, dental problems.

Eye Exam
Visual acuity

Visual acuity impairment may cause perceptual problems which the patient interprets as dizziness. New glasses may also produce perceptual problems. Cataracts cause visual impairment, and following cataract extraction the patient may experience difficulty with ambulation. Distortion of vision due to strong positive lenses produces disorientation poorly tolerated by patients with other sensory deficits.

Visual fields

Deficiency in visual fields may indicate organic lesions of the optic tract or tumor.

Extraocular movements

Decreased extraocular movements may indicate muscular weakness or damage to the 3rd, 4th or 6th cranial nerve. Diplopia, secondary to longstanding ocular muscle imbalance, produces vague lightheadedness upon gaze in the direction of diplopia.

Nystagmus

Nystagmus with vertigo is produced because of disturbances in the nervous pathway connecting vestibular nuclei with nuclei of the extrinsic muscles of the eye. Unprovoked spontaneous nystagmus is always pathological, but the significance is variable.

Vertical nystagmus (spontaneous or positional) is central in origin. It indicates bilateral brainstem disease. Synchronous horizontal nystagmus can be either central or labyrinthine in origin. Nystagmus occurring between attacks of dizziness indicates brain or cerebellopontine angle pathology. With lesions of the posterior fossa, onset of nystagmus is immediate upon assumption of a provocative position; the nystagmus does not slow or decrease in time. Nystagmus associated with benign positional vertigo (a peripheral vestibular disorder) occurs after a latent period of a few seconds following assumption of a provocative position, and slows down or decreases upon repetition of the maneuver.

Drugs such as diphenylhydantoin can also cause sustained nystagmus.

Neurological Exam
Cerebral function deficit

Indicates a more extensive central nervous system disorder such as multiple sclerosis or cerebrovascular accident.

Test the patient's intellectual function with: serial 7's, orientation, memory ability and definition of proverbs.

Cranial nerve deficit	May help to localize lesion responsible for the disorder. Presence of cranial nerve deficits, in addition to the 8th (acoustic), indicates more extensive lesions or underlying central nervous system involvement, as with vertebral and basilar artery occlusion.
Motor function	Tests should include muscle strength and range of motion, as well as gait.
	See Subjective Rationale, impaired gait (p. 144). With a cerebrovascular accident there may be unilateral weakness or paralysis. Patients with multiple sclerosis may have motor deficits. Patients with parkinsonism may interpret motor impairment as dizziness. Patients with diabetic neuropathy may have decreased motor function.
Sensory function	Decreased sensation is seen with diabetic neuropathy and sometimes with alcoholism. Specific tests to be done are position sense, light and deep touch and vibratory sense.
Cerebellar function Past pointing	With peripheral vestibular involvement, both arms will miss the original points. With central origin, one or both arms may show deficit.
Coordination tests	Deficit in fine coordination (rapid alternating movements, finger to nose tests) indicates cerebellar lesion or ischemia of basilar area.
	During the Romberg test, a patient with peripheral vestibular involve-

ment has a tendency to consistently fall toward one side. Other central nervous system diseases may also present with a positive Romberg.

Gait has been discussed previously (p. 144).

Reflexes

Deep tendon reflexes may be decreased with neuropathy.

Cardiovascular Exam

To rule out or confirm cardiovascular origin of dizziness. See Subjective Rationale for specific information. Look specifically for arrhythmias, evidence of poor circulation, bruits in vessels indicative of occlusions, carotid sinus sensitivity. Also see Vital Signs under Objective Data.

Dizziness Simulation Tests

The purpose of these tests is to reproduce the dizziness, if possible.

Change in position
Sudden turn when walking

Have the patient sit, stand, lie down, turn head or get into any position in which he has experienced dizziness.

Patients with multiple sensory deficits, especially those with peripheral neuropathy, may complain of lightheadedness when walking and making a sharp turn. A sense of position, and thus relief of the dizziness sensation, may be obtained by having the patient touch a stable object such as the examiner.

Carotid sinus stimulation

Stimulate each carotid sinus separately for 10 seconds. Must be done carefully in persons over age 60, as cerebral ischemia may result.

Hyperventilation	Have patient hyperventilate for 3 minutes. Dizziness or vertigo may only be reproducible after carrying out other positional maneuvers following hyperventilation. See Subjective Rationale on Hyperventilation.
Valsalva maneuver	Have the patient do forced expiration against closed glottis for 15 seconds. The increased intrathoracic pressure stimulates a vagal response which results in decreased cardiac output and hypoxia.
Sitting/standing with eyes open and closed	Patient may lose sense of position.
Blood pressure lying and standing	Orthostatic hypotension may be detected upon standing.
Positional vertigo maneuver	*Nylen-Barany maneuver:* The patient is abruptly moved from a sitting position to a prone position with his head hanging at a 45 degree angle and rotated first to one side and then the other. This test will be positive for vertigo/ nystagmus with vestibular disorders.

Lab Data

Urinalysis	Screening test for diabetes mellitus.
Complete blood count	Rule out anemia, infection.

Blood sugar
  Fasting or 2-hour
  postprandial
	Rule out diabetes mellitus.

Electrolytes	Indicated with suspected cardiovascular problem.

X-Rays
Cervical spine

Rule out osteophytes, spondylosis, trauma.

Skull

Rule out trauma, lesions.

Electrocardiogram (EKG)

Indicated if arrhythmias suspected, particularly heart block.

ASSESSMENT:
Benign positional vertigo

Severe rotational sensation upon abrupt change of position. Duration is brief and may be accompanied by nausea and vomiting; no hearing loss. Nystagmus and vertigo occur a few seconds after assuming the provocative position, but adaptation and fatigue occur upon repetition of the maneuver. No other neurological signs are present.

Labyrinthitis

Sudden onset of primary attack of vertigo. Accompanied by fullness in ear but no deafness or tinnitus. Cause is usually viral; recent upper respiratory infection may be in history. Course is self-limiting and disappears in a few weeks. Could be bacterial meningitis if accompanied with severe, persistent headache.

Ear infection
Otitis media
Mastoiditis

Dizziness is accompanied by fullness in ear, possibly pain. Signs of infection in ear are present: drainage, erythema, fluid. Fever may be present.

Meniere's disease

Sudden, violent onset, associated with nausea and vomiting. Duration of each episode 30 minutes to several hours. No vertigo between attacks. Accompanied by fullness in ear, tinnitus and hearing loss, which fluctuates. Hearing loss is usually unilateral and is sensorineural or inner ear type. May be free of attacks for months at a time before another occurs.

Hyperventilation

There is a history of breathlessness, anxiousness, (possibly) frontal headaches and finger and perioral paresthesia. Dizziness is chronic, episodic, without ear symptoms; dizziness can be reproduced with hyperventilation. Nystagmus on positional maneuver may be present after hyperventilating.

Multiple sensory deficits

Examination reveals two of the following: neuropathy, visual impairment, vestibular deficits, cervical spondylosis, other orthopedic disorders interfering with ambulation.

The patient with multiple sensory deficits experiences a loss of perspective in position and is unsteady when walking. The dizziness is chronic, and may be relieved merely by touching a stable object. This helps regain a sense of perspective in position.

Psychogenic dizziness

Dizziness of psychogenic origin is usually longstanding. Patient reveals history of stress, anxiety or depression. The dizziness may be associated or precipitated by hyperventilation.

Cerebrovascular disorders
  Vertebral-basilar artery
  insufficiency

Constant vertigo accompanied by syncope, headache, visual problems, ataxia, leg weakness, facial tingling or numbness and other cranial nerve deficits. The neurological findings may not present until a few weeks after the dizziness begins. Coarse nystagmus in between the dizzy spells, plus excessive imbalance, points to basilar ischemia.

Acoustic neuroma
Brain tumor

May present with unilateral hearing loss and tinnitus with constant nonsevere vertigo. May have episodes of confusion, mood changes, head pain and neurological deficits such as 5th and 7th cranial nerve abnormalities.

Cardiovascular disorders

Produce chronic, intermittent or constant dizziness. May be positional and occur immediately upon standing. This is a common cause for dizziness in the elderly. Dizziness may be present as a side-effect of antihypertensive medication, particularly alphamethyldopa and guanethidine. Syncope with carotid sinus hypersensitivity, evidence of arrhythmias and hypertension lead one to suspect cardiovascular origin of dizziness. No ear symptoms are present with cardiovascular related dizziness.

Trauma

An unsteady feeling rather than true vertigo is usually present. Cervical muscle spasms may occur. History of head or neck trauma leads one to suspect this cause.

PLAN:
Diagnostic
Further lab work
T_3/T_4

Indicated if thyroid deficiency is suspected.

Lumbar puncture

To rule out bacterial meningitis.

Consults

ENT: Indicated if ear problem present.

Neurological: Indicated with presence of abnormal neurological signs.

Orthopedic: Indicated if orthopedic problem present.

Cardiovascular: Indicated if examination reveals cardiac problems.

Psychiatric: Indicated if psychogenic origin suspected; must exclude other causes first.

Treatment

May refer patient to other clinic appropriate for problem.

Benign positional vertigo

Have patient repeatedly assume head position that precipitates vertigo; this encourages adaptation and compensation of the central nervous system. Explain that this procedure will take time.

Labyrinthitis

If viral in origin, it is self-limiting. Bed rest may be indicated until symptoms disappear, along with tranquilizer, antinausea and antivertigo medications. If lumbar puncture reveals positive bacterial culture, antibiotics are indicated for treatment and the patient must be admitted.

Ear infection

Treatment of infection will resolve the underlying problem and the dizziness and other symptoms will disappear. Referral to otolaryngology may be indicated.

Meniere's disease

Referral to otolaryngology is necessary for further audiometric tests. There is no universally accepted treatment for this disease. The patient suffers extreme physical and psychological stress and thus needs much support. Stressful situations may precipitate crises and counseling may be helpful. Discontinue use of alcohol and smoking to decrease stimulation of the sympathetic nervous system. Tranquilizers may be of help as is a low-salt diet (the physiological effect of this is questionable; originally thought that reducing the sodium ion would affect the increased endolymph fluid in the labyrinth). Reassurance that this is not a fatal disease is most important.

Hyperventilation

Underlying condition causing hyperventilation must be corrected. Most often emotional stress is cause of this overbreathing. Identification of the stress and helping to cope with or eliminate it is necessary for treatment. Rebreathing into a paper bag may abort the acute attack.

Multiple sensory deficits

Referral to appropriate clinic is indicated.

Psychogenic problem

Counseling and perhaps referral for psychiatric help is necessary.

Cerebrovascular disorders

Referral to Neurology indicated.

Acoustic neuroma Brain tumors	Referral to Neurology indicated.
Cardiovascular disorders	Referral to Cardiology indicated.
Trauma	Treatment depends on the injury. Referral to appropriate clinic and care as indicated.
Patient education	Dizziness or vertigo can be very incapacitating, or merely a bothersome problem. In either case, the patient needs much reassurance. To reassure the patient that he does not have a brain tumor (if this is proven by exam and tests) is essential, as this may be an unverbalized fear. Stress may be the underlying cause for dizziness. Dizziness as yet undiagnosed can cause stress for the patient; therefore, much understanding and support is needed. Any information regarding exam, tests and treatment may help relieve the stress. Other education may include instructing the patient to assume different positions slowly, or to steady himself by using handrails, furniture or another person as a guide while walking. Hyperventilation can be very frightening and instruction on how to stop the sequence of hyperventilation may be necessary.

BIBLIOGRAPHY

Clairmont, Albert A., John S. Turner Jr., and Richard T. Jackson: "Dizziness, A Logical Approach to Diagnosis and Treatment," *Postgraduate Medicine,* vol. 56, no. 2, pp. 139–144, August 1974.

Conn, Howard F., and Rex B. Conn Jr., (eds.): *Current Diagnosis 4,* Philadelphia: Saunders, 1974.

Drachman, David A., and Cecil W. Hart: "An Approach to the Dizzy Patient," *Neurology*, vol. 22, no. 4, pp. 323–334, April 1972.

Elia, Joseph Charles, M.D.: *The Dizzy Patient*, Springfield, Illinois: Charles C Thomas Publisher, 1968.

Fisher, C. M.: "Vertigo in Cerebrovascular Disease," *Archives of Otolaryngology*, vol. 85, pp. 529–534, May 1967.

MacBryde, C. M. (ed.): *Signs and Symptoms*, 5th ed., Philadelphia: Lippincott, pp. 723–745, 1970.

Merifield, David O.: "Self Limited Idiopathic Vertigo (Epidemic Vertigo)," *Archives of Otolaryngology*, vol. 81, pp. 355–358, 1965.

Saunders, William H.: "Meniere's Disease: A Dizzying Ringing Maelstrom," *Modern Medicine*, pp. 20–24, July 8, 1974.

Singer, Ellis P.: "The Hyperventilation Syndrome in Clinical Medicine," *New York Journal of Medicine*, vol. 58, pp. 1494–1500, 1958.

Spector, Martin (ed.): *Dizziness and Vertigo: Diagnosis and Treatment*, New York: Grune and Stratton, 1967.

Weiss, Alfred D.: "Neurological Aspects of the Differential Diagnosis of Vertigo," *Annals of Otology, Rhinology and Laryngology*, vol. 77, pp. 216–221, 1968.

NOTES

NOTES

Chapter 8

Dysuria

DYSURIA WORKSHEET

To be used for patients with:
Bladder/Kidney Infection
Penile Discharge
Burning with Urination
Venereal Disease

What you can't afford to miss: pyelonephritis, gonorrhea.

Chief Complaint: _____
SUBJECTIVE DATA:

DESCRIBE POSITIVE RESPONSES
(Include Onset, Severity, Duration, Location)
Yes　　*No*

___　___　Frequency: _____

___　___　Urgency: _____

___　___　Trouble starting or decreasing force of stream: _____

　　　　　_____

___　___　Genital itching/burning: _____

___ ___ Nocturia: _____

___ ___ Hematuria: _____

___ ___ Foul-smelling urine: _____

___ ___ Cloudy urine:_____

___ ___ Abdominal pain: _____

___ ___ Back pain: _____

___ ___ Fever/chills: _____

___ ___ Penile/vaginal discharge:

                Color: _____

                Amount: _____

___ ___ Genital sore(s):

                Location:_____

___ ___ Painful

___ ___ Rash:_____

___ ___ Dyspareunia: _____

___ ___ Stress incontinence:

                Gravida: _____

                Para:_____

                AB: _____

___ ___ Pregnant:

                LMP: _____

—— —— Previous UTI's:

        Number: _____

        Treatment: _____

        Previous evaluation: _____

—— —— Previous NSU:

        Number: _____

        Treatment: _____

—— —— Previous V.D.:

        Type: _____

        Treatment: _____

—— —— Diabetes:

        Date: _____

        Treatment: _____

—— —— Hypertension:

        Date: _____

        Treatment: _____

—— —— Renal calculi:

        Date: _____

        Treatment: _____

—— —— Allergies (list allergen and reaction):

_____

_____

___ ___ Medications (specify):

_____

_____

OBJECTIVE DATA:

Vital signs: _____B/P _____P _____T _____Wt

DESCRIBE POSITIVE RESPONSES

Yes   No

___ ___ Penile/vaginal discharge: _____

___ ___ Sores/warts:_____

___ ___ Rash:_____

___ ___ Inguinal nodes:_____

___ ___ CVA tenderness: _____

PELVIC EXAM: _____Not Done

Yes   No

___ ___ External genitalia reddened: _____

___ ___ Urethra red/swollen/discharge: _____

___ ___ Vulvar lesions: _____

___ ___ Cystocele/rectocele: _____

___ ___ Vaginal lesion: _____

___ ___ Cervical erosion: _____

___ ___ Cervical tenderness: _____

___ ___ Uterine enlargement/tenderness: _____

___ ___ Mass/fullness: _____

___ ___ Adnexal tenderness/fullness: _____

___ ___ Other: _____

MALE EXAM: _____Not Done
Yes   No

___ ___ Scrotum enlarged/tender: _____

___ ___ Scrotal mass: _____

___ ___ Prostate enlarged/tender: _____

___ ___ Other: _____

LAB DATA:
Done Not
      Done

___ ___ Wet prep:

_____Yeast

_____Trichomonas

_____Increased bacteria

_____Negative

___ ___ Urinalysis:

_____WBC

_____RBC

_____Bacteria

_____Casts

_____pH

_____Blood

_____Bilirubin

_____Acetone

_____Protein

_____Glucose

___ ___ GC. smear:

_____Positive

_____Negative:

___ ___ Pregnancy test:

_____Positive

_____Negative

___ ___ Darkfield:

_____Positive

_____Negative

___ ___ 3-glass urine:

Results: _____

ASSESSMENT:

_____

_____

_____

_____

PLAN:
DIAGNOSTIC:

_____Urine C & S

_____GC. culture:

_____Cx

_____Vag.

_____Urethral

_____Rectal

_____Pharynx

_____Viral culture

_____Serologies:

_____VDRL

_____FTA

_____Viral

_____Other tests: _____

_____Consult: _____

THERAPEUTIC:

_____Admit: _____

_____Medications (Specify): _____

_____

_____Other: _____

171

PATIENT EDUCATION:

_____Return in 2 days if symptoms persist

_____Return for urine reculture 1 week after completing antibiotic therapy

_____Call in 2 days for GC. culture results

_____Return in 1 week for GC. reculture (if treated today)

_____Medication instructions: _____

_____

_____Other (specify): _____

_____

DYSURIA WORKSHEET RATIONALE

SUBJECTIVE DATA:

Frequency

May be present as a result of an inability to empty the bladder due to urethral spasms resulting from an inflammation of the trigone area (trigonitis). True frequency must be differentiated from frequency due to nonpathologic causes such as increased fluid intake or anxiety.

Urgency

Also related to spasms at the site of the trigone.

Trouble starting or decreasing force of stream

Due to urethral obstruction, usually prostatic. Poor bladder muscle tone, neurogenic or from overdistention, may cause this also.

Genital itching or burning	Skin irritation resulting from vaginal discharge may cause itching and burning with urination. Patient usually describes this as "burning on the outside." True dysuria results from urethral irritation.
Nocturia	Confirms true frequency when this finding is a change for the patient.
Hematuria	Indicative of a pathologic process in the urinary tract. Vaginal contamination must be ruled out.
Foul-smelling urine	May be produced by bacterial activity.
Cloudy urine	Produced by the presence of abnormal elements such as bacteria, casts, cells and amorphous debris. Phosphates are normal precipitants, especially in early-morning specimens that have been allowed to stand.
Abdominal pain	Suprapubic or lower abdominal pain usually indicates lower urinary tract disease or bladder inflammation.
Back pain	Pain in the area of the costovertebral angle indicates kidney inflammation and upper urinary tract disease.
Fever and chills	Indicate a systemic process and usually relates to upper urinary tract disease.
Penile discharge	Nonspecific urethritis and gonorrhea may be associated with dysuria either with or without discharge.

Vaginal discharge

Skin irritation resulting from vaginal discharge may cause "burning with urination." Recent data also suggest an association between exacerbations of vaginitis/cervicitis and bacterial colonization of the introitus and urethra.

Genital sore

History of indurated, nontender lesion on the genitalia makes one suspect chancre. Painful ulcerations can occur with vaginal discharge or herpes II infection. Condyloma acuminatum (venereal wart) presents as painless "bump."

Rash

Rash of secondary syphilis usually appears 6-8 weeks after the chancre. It is widespread, involving face, palms and soles, is rarely pruritic; lesions are usually maculopapular or pustular, although there can be great variation in the appearance of the rash. The rash of gonococcemia most commonly occurs on the lower extremities, and is papular, petechial or associated with hemorrhagic pustules.

Dyspareunia

Frequently associated with vaginitis or cervicitis.

Stress incontinence

Loss of pelvic muscle tone frequently accompanies multiple pregnancies. Multiparity may also cause loss of the normal angle at the bladder neck and urethra allowing bacteria easier access to the bladder.

Pregnant
   Last menstrual period

Pregnancy will influence choice of drug treatment and decision about radiographic evaluation, if indicated. Pregnancy may predispose to urinary tract infection through compression of the ureters and interference with urine flow by the enlarging uterus.

Previous urinary tract
infections

Include age at onset, site, organism, sensitivities, antibiotic therapy and follow-up cultures. A history of documented, recurrent UTI's requires thorough evaluation, including cystoscopy and intravenous pyelogram, to determine the etiology.

Previous nonspecific
urethritis
Previous venereal disease

May give clue to present problem if symptoms and findings are similar to past problem.

History of diabetes/
   hypertension/renal calculi

Urinary tract infections, particularly pyelonephritis, are more common in these individuals. In the diabetic, this may be related to bladder dysfunction and alterations in cellular and humoral defense mechanisms.

Allergies

Will influence choice of treatment.

Medications

May influence choice of treatment; may also affect test results, if, for example, patient recently took antibiotics. Recent douching or use of vaginal medications will invalidate wet prep findings; use of acetylsalicylic acid within last 24 hours will invalidate some pregnancy test results.

OBJECTIVE DATA:

Blood pressure, pulse, temperature

Provide data on general status. Fever may indicate inflammatory/infectious process.

Penile/vaginal discharge

See under Subjective Data.

Sores/warts

Syphilitic chancre is a painless, indurated lesion with raised borders. Herpes simplex II lesions are vesicular or ulcerative and may be secondarily infected. Small ulcerations may also occur due to irritation from vaginal discharge. Venereal warts are cauliflower-like projections arising from a pedicle; the condyloma latum of syphilis is wart-like and flat.

Rash

See Subjective Data.

Inguinal Nodes

Are enlarged and tender in infectious processes of the genitalia or pelvis.

Costovertebral angle tenderness

May indicate upper urinary tract inflammation.

Pelvic Exam
External genitalia (urethra, vulva)

Evaluated for redness, edema, presence of discharge and lesions, since this may be the cause of burning with urination.

Cystocele, rectocele

May contribute to obstruction and stasis with resulting urinary infection.

Cervical erosion/tenderness

Usually associated with vaginitis and cervicitis. Pelvic pain upon movement of the cervix may indicate upward extension of an infectious process.

Uterine enlargement/ tenderness/mass	May be associated with pregnancy or pelvic inflammatory disease.
Adnexal tenderness/ fullness/mass	May indicate upward spread of an inflammatory process into the fallopian tubes. May also be associated with tumor, cyst or abscess.

Male Exam

Scrotum enlarged/ tender/mass	May be due to orchitis or epididymitis from gonococci or other organisms.
Prostate enlarged, tender	May be the site of an infectious process. A tender prostate should *not* be massaged as this may lead to sepsis.

Lab Data

Wet prep	Performed on vaginal discharge to rule out monilial or trichomonal vaginitis and nonspecific vaginitis. See Vaginal Discharge Protocol for procedure.
Urinalysis	A clean catch specimen is obtained in the following manner:

Instruct woman to clean the urethra with green soap and warm water using 3 separate sponges (each used only once with a downward motion). The labia should be spread with the fingers and a midstream sample obtained.

The urine should be examined microscopically immediately for white blood cells, red blood cells, bacteria, crystals or casts. If there will be a delay in plating it for culture, it should be refrigerated. Gram-negative bacteria have a doubling time of 20 minutes at room temperature; thus contaminants may overgrow, especially in samples taken from women with vaginal discharges. Microscopic examination of the unspun urine will reveal organisms in 70 % of patients with greater than 100,000 organisms/ml.

Pyuria, defined as 3-5 WBC's per high power field, will usually be present if the patient is symptomatic, but will only be present in 40 % of patients when they have asymptomatic bacteriuria.

Gonorrhea smear

Performed on urethral discharge in males to rule out the presence of gram-negative intracellular diplococci. Smears in females are not as accurate due to the presence of other forms of Neisseria in the normal vaginal flora.

Pregnancy test

Usually performed if at least 6 weeks after last normal menses. Some medications, notably acetylsalicylic acid, may give a false positive result if taken within the past 24 hours.

Darkfield

Performed on discharge from suspected chancre to identify presence of spirochetes.

3-glass urine specimen

In males, there is some value in separating out the stream to determine what is from the urethra and prostate and what is from the bladder. This is done by obtaining a 3-glass urine test. The patient must void *without interruption* into 3 separate containers. The initial specimen contains contents from the anterior urethra; the midstream urine represents bladder contents; the terminal specimen may contain sediment from the prostate and seminal vesicles.

ASSESSMENT:

Some of the more common conditions associated with dysuria are:

Urinary Tract Infection
Cystitis

Usually produces dysuria, frequency, urgency, pain in lower back or lower abdomen and low-grade fever. Urine may be cloudy or odorous; gross hematuria occurs with acute hemorrhagic cystitis. Urinalysis shows pyuria, bacteriuria, hematuria and often proteinuria. The infection usually responds to a sulfonamide. Recurrent attacks may lead to pyelonephritis and require a full urologic evaluation.

Acute pyelonephritis

Associated with fever, shaking chills, malaise, flank pain, costovertebral angle tenderness, dysuria and leukocytosis. May follow lower urinary tract infection. Urinalysis shows pyuria, bacteriuria, hematuria, proteinuria and casts. Antibiotics are prescribed on the basis of urine culture and sensitivity findings.

Recurrent infections require a thorough evaluation and prolonged follow-up.

Chronic pyelonephritis

May be asymptomatic or present with picture of acute pyelonephritis. There is usually a history of recurrent or chronic urinary tract infections. Urinalysis may show findings similar to acute pyelonephritis, but on an intermittent basis. Obstruction is a major predisposing factor and cystoscopy and intravenous pyelogram should be done to rule out a surgically correctable lesion. Long-term antibiotic therapy is usually required.

Gonorrhea

The causative organism is *Neisseria gonorrhoeae*. Transmission is by sexual contact with an average incubation period of 3-5 days. Symptoms of dysuria, urgency and urethral discharge are common in the male, although asymptomatic male carriers exist. A significant number of infected females are asymptomatic. In males, the diagnosis is established by visualization of the intracellular gram-negative diplococcus in the urethral discharge. Smears of vaginal discharge are unreliable due to the normal presence of other Neisseria forms; therefore, culture on Thayer-Martin medium is required for diagnosis in the female.

Penicillin is the treatment of choice.

See Vaginal Discharge Protocol for additional information.

Nonspecific Urethritis (NSU)

Usually presents with low-grade urethritis, scanty to moderate mucopurulent urethral discharge and dysuria of varying degree. Diagnosis is made by exclusion of *Neisseria gonorrhoeae*. Implicated organisms include mycoplasma, mixed bacteria, Trichomonas, *Candida albicans* and the bedsonia group. Chronic prostatitis may be a complication.

NSU does not respond to penicillin; tetracycline is probably the most effective treatment choice. Relapse is common and some advocate treating the sexual partner in recurrent cases.

Prostatitis
Acute

The prostate will be enlarged and tender. Large mucus shreds appear in the terminal specimen of a 3-glass urine test. The prostate should *not* be massaged to obtain fluid for examination as sepsis may result.

Chronic

Prostatic palpation may reveal normal findings. With a history of chronic urinary tract infection, the 3-glass urine test should be performed; a positive test will reveal large mucus shreds in the terminal specimen. Prostatic massage usually expresses fluid containing many leukocytes. Treatment is often unsatisfactory; broad spectrum antibiotics are indicated after urological consultation.

Reiter's Syndrome

Classically presents with the triad of urethritis, arthritis and conjunctivitis. Occurs most frequently in young males, with the acute

181

episode subsiding spontaneously after several weeks. Urethritis usually precedes the onset of the other findings and often does not respond to antibiotics. Important diagnostic features include the associated skin, mucous membrane and ocular lesions as well as the asymmetrical arthritis. The underlying joint inflammation usually requires primary management. Recent data suggest that a bedsonia or Chlamydia infection may cause the syndrome.

PLAN:

Diagnostic

Urine culture and sensitivity

To identify specific causative organisms and their antibiotic sensitivity in order to initiate appropriate treatment.

The urine culture evaluation is crucial. Greater than 100,000 organisms/ml. is the figure accepted as the most reliable indicator of significant bacteriuria. However, it is a statistical figure and only 95 % of patients with significant bacteriuria will have 100,000 organisms/ml. in a single specimen. Virtually 100 % of patients will have that number of organisms if 3 consecutive specimens were to be obtained. The count may be lower if the patient has been on antibiotics or has taken a water load before being seen.

Gram-negative rods may be significant in concentrations less than 100,000 organisms/ml.; enterococci are also significant in lower concentration. Diphtheroids, *S. epidermidis,* lactobacilli, micrococcus and S. *viridans* almost never have any significance when found in urine, as they are usually contaminants. Some patients may not have bacteria in their urine but a viral culture may be positive to indicate a probable viral urinary tract infection.

Sensitivities should be requested on all organisms.

Gonorrhea cultures (from cervix in females; from urethra in males)

Should be plated on Thayer-Martin medium and chocolate agar. Rectal and pharyngeal cultures may provide additional information in selected patients, e.g. homosexual males.

Viral culture if perineal and/or pelvic lesions

To determine the presence of herpes simplex virus type II. This has implications for patient education regarding the frequency of pap smears and pregnancy. See Vaginal Discharge Protocol.

Serologies

VDRL and FTA are performed to rule out syphilis. If suspected herpetic lesions are present, a viral serology should be done.

Other tests
Consult

There is some feeling that an initial urinary tract infection in a male warrants an intravenous pyelogram and Urology referral as this is most likely an upper urinary tract problem. Likewise, after 2 documented urinary tract infections in a female, one should consider intravenous pyelogram and cystoscopy to identify lower urinary tract pathology.

Therapeutic
Admit

Admit patients with pyelonephritis if pregnant, if there is a complicating illness or if they appear septic. Ideally, all patients with pyelonephritis should be admitted for 24 hour observation.

Medications

For first infections, a sulfonamide is usually effective.

For patients with a history of previous urinary tract infections, the previous sensitivity of the organisms should be checked. If felt that this is a relapse, the organism should be treated accordingly. If thought to be a reinfection in a young female, a sulfonamide may again be sufficient for treatment. Some might recommend ampicillin in this situation.

Any concurrent vaginitis should be appropriately treated. See Vaginal Discharge Protocol.

Patient education
and follow-up
For urinary tract infection

1. The patient should be rechecked in 48 hours if still symptomatic. At that time sensitivities will be available and another antimicrobial can be chosen if necessary.

2. If the patient is asymptomatic he should be told to return for reculture in 1 week after completing therapy.

3. Ideally, urine should be recultured at the end of 2 months even if it is negative at the 2-3 week

check. If negative again at 2 months, the patient should be instructed to return only if symptoms recur.

4. If the urinary tract infection is related to sexual intercourse, the patient should be advised to void after intercourse. In some patients who have recurrent UTI despite postcoital voiding, an antibacterial is sometimes given. For example, sulfa or penicillin G at the time of intercourse and 8 or 12 hours later.

For gonorrhea

The patient should be instructed to call for the results of the gonorrhea culture in 2 days and return for treatment if the culture is positive.

Medications

Specific instructions should be given regarding the proper regimen for taking medication, expected results and side effects.

BIBLIOGRAPHY

Harvey, A. McGehee, et al. (eds): *The Principles and Practice of Medicine,* New York: Appleton-Century-Crofts, 1972.

Houston, J. C., C. L. Joiner, and J. R. Trounce: *A Short Textbook of Medicine,* 4th ed., London: English Universities Press LTD, 1972.

"Nonspecific Urethritis," *Medical Clinics of North America,* vol. 56, no. 5, pp. 1193–1202, September 1972.

Chapter 9

Headache

HEADACHE WORKSHEET

> To be used in patients with:
> Headache
> Pressure in Head

> **What you can't afford to miss: meningitis, intracranial bleeding, temporal arteritis.**

Chief Complaint:_____

SUBJECTIVE DATA:

Location: _____

Duration: _____

Frequency: _____

Course: _____

Radiation: _____

Character: _____

Precipitated by:_____

Made worse by: _____

Relieved by: _____

Onset: _____

DESCRIBE POSITIVE RESPONSES
(Include Onset, Severity, Duration)

ASSOCIATED WITH:

Yes   No

___ ___ Previous similar symptoms: _____

___ ___ Altered mental status:_____

___ ___ Prodrome or aura: _____

___ ___ Related to menses: _____

___ ___ Trauma: _____Date _____Type

___ ___ Loss of consciousness: _____

___ ___ Rhinorrhea:_____

___ ___ Nausea:_____

___ ___ Vomiting:_____

___ ___ Seizures: _____

___ ___ Local disease:

_____Dental caries/abscess:_____

_____Sinusitis: _____

_____Otitis/mastoiditis: _____

_____Neck pain/stiffness: _____

_____Nasal stuffiness: _____

189

___ ___ Ocular symptoms:

     _____Tearing: _____

     _____Photophobia: _____

     _____Blurry vision:_____

     _____Scotomata: _____

___ ___ Systemic symptoms:

     _____Chills/fever/sweats:_____

     _____Myalgia: _____

     _____Weight loss: _____

     _____Anxiety or stress in life:_____

___ ___ Past history:

     _____Birth control pills: _____

     _____Other medicines: _____

     _____Significant past illnesses: _____

     _____Allergies:_____

     _____Family history of migraine: _____

     _____Other: _____

OBJECTIVE DATA:
    General: _____B/P _____P _____R _____T

    General appearance and affect: _____

    Sex: _____Male _____Female

DESCRIBE POSITIVE RESPONSES

HEAD EXAM: _____Not Done

Yes   No

____ ____ Meningismus

____ ____ Local tenderness (head and neck):

Location: _____

Degree: _____

____ ____ Teeth abnormal: _____

____ ____ External eyes abnormal: _____

____ ____ Fundi abnormal: _____

____ ____ Ear pathology: _____

NEUROLOGICAL EXAMINATION—(explain if abnormal): _____Not Done

Abnormal   Normal

_____ _____ Mental status:

Orientation: _____

Serial 7's: _____

_____ _____ Cranial nerves: _____

_____ _____ Deep tendon reflexes (grade 0-4+): _____

_____

_____ _____ Plantar reflex: _____

_____ _____ Motor strength: _____

_____ _____ Gait: _____

_____ _____ Romberg: _____

Protocols for Common Acute Self-Limiting Problems

_____ _____ Finger-to-nose

_____ _____ Sensory:

Light touch: _____

Pinprick: _____

_____ _____ Speech: _____

LAB DATA:
Done Not
Done

___ ___ CBC: _____

___ ___ ESR: _____

___ ___ Sinus x-rays: _____

___ ___ Dental x-rays: _____

___ ___ Skull x-rays: _____

___ ___ Lumbar puncture: _____

ASSESSMENT:

_____ Tension headache

_____ Migraine—common
—classic

_____ Cluster headache

_____ Sinusitis

_____ Hypertensive headache

_____ Suspect brain tumor

_____ Meningitis

_____ Intracranial bleeding

_____ Traumatic or post-traumatic headache

_____ Temporal arteritis

_____ Other (specify): _____

PLAN:

_____ Admission: _____

_____ Neurology consult or referral: _____

Date:_____

_____ Other clinic or referral (e.g. medical, psychiatric):

_____

DIAGNOSTIC:

_____Electroencephalogram

_____Brain scan

THERAPEUTIC:

_____Analgesic: _____

_____Decongestant: _____

_____Tranquilizer: _____

_____Ergot preparation: _____

_____Steroids: _____

_____Antibiotics:_____

_____Antihypertensive:_____

_____Other: _____

PATIENT EDUCATION:

_____Medication instruction and explanation:_____

_____

_____Explanation of further studies: _____

_____

_____Call for test results:_____

_____Return appointment: _____

_____Symptoms to return for:_____

_____Situational stress:_____

_____Other: _____

HEADACHE WORKSHEET RATIONALE

SUBJECTIVE DATA:

Location

Bilateral
Generalized

Occipital-nuchal in tension headache with radiation over entire cranium.

Classically is occipital in hypertension, usually with diastolic greater than 120 mm. Hg.

Pain with meningitis and subarachnoid hemorrhage may be local or generalized.

Found in post-traumatic headache.

Unilateral or localized	Usually characteristic of migraine, cluster, tumor or sinus headaches.
	Temporal arteritis is usually localized to area of the disease process or to one side of the head.
	Typical of headache due to glaucoma.
Duration	Tension headaches are usually gradual in onset and may last hours to weeks to months.
	Hypertensive headaches usually worse on awakening and improve as day progresses.
	Common migraine lasts several days.
	Classic migraine usually lasts less than 24 hours.
	Cluster headache awakens patient and may last several hours.
	Sinus headache lasts hours to days.
	Headache due to tumor intermittent to constant, may be worse in the morning.
Frequency *Course*	This is quite variable.
	Tension headaches may occur daily or be constant for days. They may not recur for several weeks or months.
	Vascular headaches (migraine, cluster) tend to occur in clusters. The

patient will have a great deal of trouble for a few weeks or months and then may be pain-free for months or years. The reason for this pattern is unclear.

The frequency of the headache of sinusitis, tumor, subdural, etc., is related to the underlying disease.

Radiation

Usually not helpful in distinguishing various types of headaches.

Character/Intensity

The headache of migraine and hypertension may be throbbing. Tension, muscular and sinus headaches may be described as band-like pressure.

A steady aching headache is seen with brain tumor.

Precipitated by, Made Worse by

Tension headache is usually related to stress or depression.

Hypertensive headache is obviously related to increased blood pressure.

Common migraine headache may be triggered by stress. There is usually a family history of migraine.

Classic migraine may be aggravated by noise or light. It is more frequent during pregnancy or may be associated with birth control pills. There is usually a family history.

Cluster headache usually has onset 2-3 hours after going to sleep. More common in spring and fall.

Relieved by	Vascular headaches, especially cluster headaches, may be better in the upright position. Lying down helps sinus and tension headaches. Analgesia may help all headaches, but vascular headaches are often refractory to the common analgesics.
Onset	Headache due to subarachnoid bleeding occurs very suddenly secondary to arterial bleeding. Headache due to vascular causes or meningitis can be very rapid in onset.

Associated with

Previous similar symptoms	Previous diagnosis or symptoms may give insight into the present problem.
Altered mental status	Tension headaches may be associated with depression. With migraine headache, the patient may be dejected, withdrawn or listless.
	Altered orientation or behavior change may be seen with organic lesions.
Prodrome or aura	Usually visual. Unilateral numbness may be seen with vascular headaches secondary to initial arterial spasm and local ischemia in the area affected.
Relation to menses	Vascular headaches may occur just prior to onset of menstruation. The role of fluid retention in this situation is unclear.
Trauma Loss of consciousness	A strong history of these events would suggest intracranial bleeding

	(e.g. subdural) or "post-traumatic" headache.
Rhinorrhea	Purulent rhinorrhea suggests sinusitis and the possibility of associated bacterial meningitis.
	Cerebrospinal fluid (CSF) rhinorrhea is diagnostic of skull fracture with CSF leak.
Nausea, vomiting	Associated with any severe headache, but may occur with little or no headache in migraine. Vomiting without nausea may occur in tumor headache.
Seizures	Imply an organic lesion.

Local Disease

Dental caries/abscess	Causes irritation of 2nd and 3rd divisions of the trigeminal nerves, especially when upper teeth involved.
Sinusitis	May cause frontal headache; usually unilateral or bilateral due to increased pressure in sinuses. This is especially true in frontal or sphenoid sinusitis.
Otitis/mastoiditis	Infection in these areas may cause referred pain.
Neck pain/stiffness	Muscle spasm or cervical osteoarthritis may cause headache. It is usually occipital, bilateral and secondary to spasm or nerve root involvement.
Nasal stuffiness	Associated with cluster headache, nasal or paranasal disease.

Ocular Symptoms
Tearing/redness

May be seen in glaucoma or cluster headache.

Photophobia

Seen in meningitis, migraine and eye disease such as iritis or uveitis. The mechanism is unknown.

Blurred vision

Temporal arteritis may present with sudden blindness. With migraine one may get hemianopsia secondary to arterial spasm and subsequent ischemia. Ocular disease (uveitis, iritis) causes clouding of aqueous or vitreous humors.

Scotomata

Usually occurs with prodrome of migraine.

Systemic Symptoms
Chills/fever/sweats
Myalgia

May be a sign of acute infectious disease such as typhoid, rickettsial disease or viral meningitis.

Weight loss

May reflect underlying neoplasm with metastatic disease. May also reflect depression.

Anxiety or stress/
fatigability

These may be seen in tension or post-traumatic headaches. Investigation of these symptoms helps identify situational stresses which may contribute to or produce the headache.

Past History
Birth control pills

May be related to migraine headache, possibly because of the periodic withdrawal of exogenous progestogens.

Medications
(analgesic type)

May give clue to severity and how headache has affected "quality of life," especially in regard to what medications have been used, and in what quantity.

Significant past illnesses

May be related to present problem as cause of stress and anxiety. Present problem may also be direct extension of illness such as tumor, vasculitis, collagen disease, etc.

Allergies

Important in sinus disease and in planning therapeutic program.

Family history

May help diagnose migraine, as the family history is often positive in these diseases.

OBJECTIVE DATA:
Vital signs
  Blood pressure

Hypertension may be a cause of headache or can be secondary to increased intracranial pressure.

Pulse

Pulse may be increased with anxiety, either due to the pain of the headache, or secondary to anxiety about the headache. A slow pulse is seen with increased intracranial pressure.

Respirations

These may be increased with anxiety. Hypoventilation is seen with severe increased intracranial pressure as a premorbid event.

Temperature

Fever is an indication of meningitis, encephalitis or headache associated with systemic infection. Fever may also be seen in temporal arteritis and subarachnoid hemorrhage.

General appearance

A quick and general evaluation of the patient's overall condition is mandatory. An obviously severely ill individual (high fever, disoriented, in shock, lethargic or comatose) must be quickly evaluated for increased central nervous system pressure and/or infection.

Sex

Common migraine more common in women. Cluster headache almost always in men.

Head Exam
Meningismus

Indication of meningitis or subarachnoid hemorrhage. Irritation of the meninges causes reflex spasm of the neck muscles.

Neck muscle soreness and stiffness can be seen with some viral illnesses.

Local tenderness
head and neck

Present over temporal arteries in temporal arteritis.

Sinus tenderness suggests sinusitis.

Pain in cervical muscles is usually due to muscle spasm; cervical myalgia is often associated with viral illnesses or cervical spine disease.

Dental abnormalities

Severe caries or abscess may cause referred pain.

External eyes (abnormal)
Fundi (abnormal)

Look for the red eye that may be a sign of iritis or acute glaucoma which is associated with photophobia and mid-dilated pupil. Papilledema is a sign of increased intracranial pressure.

Ear pathology

Mastoid tenderness with evidence of or a history of chronic otitis media suggests mastoiditis. This may occasionally be complicated by a brain abscess.

Blood behind drum or Battles's sign (mastoid ecchymosis) implies basilar skull fracture.

Neurological Examination

Important in evaluating organic causes of headache. You are looking for generalized or focal abnormalities that may be an indication of an organic lesion. In most common headaches, the neurologic examination is normal.

Mental status

Disorientation, poor performance on serial 7's (use serial 3's if more appropriate to education) imply organic disease rather than psychiatric condition.

Cranial nerves

Abnormalities may be clue to intracranial lesions and their specific locations.

Deep tendon reflexes
Plantar reflex

Abnormalities here, often with lateralizing signs, help pinpoint location of organic lesion, e.g. bleeding, tumor; increased reflexes imply an upper motor neuron lesion.

Motor strength

The degree and symmetry of strength may give a clue to an underlying organic process. Unfortunately this is not an entirely objective part of the examination (e.g. in the malingering patient).

Gait, Romberg Finger to nose	If peripheral nerve lesions are ruled out, abnormalities here indicate a lesion in the posterior fossa.
Sensory exam	Like the motor exam, this is not entirely objective. However, with a cooperative patient, deficits here can be used to pinpoint the area of the nervous system that is abnormal.
Speech	Abnormalities of speech (e.g. slurring) may be due to specific organic lesions or may be secondary to medication (e.g. narcotics). In either case, this warrants further investigation.

Lab Data

CBC	An increased white blood count may be seen in infection or with severe stress such as subarachnoid bleeding.

Lymphocytosis may be indicative of a viral illness. |
Erythrocyte sedimentation rate	Will be elevated in most inflammatory illnesses. It is extremely high in temporal arteritis.
Dental and sinus x-ray	Will indicate pathology in these areas.
Skull x-rays	May reveal cranial or intracranial disease such as fracture, calcification, or deviation of the pineal gland secondary to a mass.

Lumbar puncture

Diagnostic in meningitis; spinal fluid will show a moderate to marked increase in white blood cells.

Sugar is decreased in infection and some tumors.

Elevated protein is seen in a wide variety of conditions and warrants further work-up.

In subarachnoid hemorrhage the fluid will show blood and xanthochromia. This procedure is contraindicated in the presence of papilledema as brainstem herniation may occur.

ASSESSMENT:

Consists of trying to fit the data obtained in the history, physical and laboratory evaluation into a diagnostic category. Some of the more common conditions are outlined below.

Tension headache

This is one of the most common types of headache and is often used as a "waste basket" term when the patient's headache cannot be given another diagnosis. Classic tension headaches are occipital-nuchal in location and are possibly produced by sustained muscular contraction in these areas. They are gradual in onset with radiation over the entire cranium and are almost always bilateral. They are sometimes associated with anxiety and depression and may last continuously for several weeks.

Hypertensive headache

Classically these headaches are present on awakening in the morning, are occipital, bilateral and tend to subside as the day progresses. They are usually associated with significant hypertension: diastolic blood pressures over 120 mm. Hg.

Common migraine

These are more common in women and usually have an onset in late adolescence or early adult life; they tend to occur following stress. They can be less frequent during pregnancy. There is usually a family history of headaches of a similar type. Common migraine can be present bilaterally and last for several days.

Classic migraine

Again, this has a strong familial predisposition, and may occur in people with personalities described as ambitious and rigid. Aura such as scotomata are common, as are sensory or motor symptoms, and there may be aggravation by noise and light. The pain is severe and unilateral, associated with nausea and vomiting and will last less than 24 hours. It is more frequent during pregnancy and may be associated with oral contraceptive use.

Cluster headache

These headaches occur almost exclusively in adult males and a family history is *not* common. Clusters tend to occur in the spring or fall and commonly awaken the patient from sleep after 2-3 hours. The headache will be unilateral, associated with tearing, redness of the eyes and nasal stuffiness. The headache usually lasts less than 2 hours.

Sinus headache

Commonly, this headache follows upper respiratory infections and is often associated with nasal or post-nasal drainage and tenderness over the affected sinus. Transillumination of the maxillary sinuses may be helpful in diagnosis.

Brain tumor headache

Classically, this headache remains localized but not necessarily over the tumor. It will often be worse in the morning and be associated with projectile vomiting. In an adult, any new headache that is severe and persistent for over 1-2 weeks requires further evaluation for this possibility. Neurologic signs will also suggest tumor, although transient focal signs can be seen with migraine and cluster headaches.

Trigeminal neuralgia

Although not truly a headache, it is characterized by recurring episodes of severe facial pain that is often brought on by moving or touching certain trigger points on the face.

Subdural hematoma

This condition almost always presents with headache as one of its manifestations with development of cranial nerve palsies. A history of trauma in the recent or distant past is common.

Post-traumatic

This is a syndrome that occurs after head trauma and is a complex consisting of giddiness, fatigability, insomnia, nervousness, trembling, irritability and inability to concentrate, in addition to severe headaches. The severity of the headache may bear no relationship to the injury.

The following types of headaches are true emergencies and must be diagnosed and treated quickly:

Bacterial meningitis and subarachnoid hemorrhage

These may have an explosive onset, particularly with hemorrhage. They are associated with stiff neck, tachycardia, fever and severe headache. The patient is usually severely ill and the need for immediate treatment is obvious.

Temporal arteritis

This condition usually appears in older people and the headache generally begins over the temporal arteries. Attacks may last for several weeks and be associated with blurring of vision and diplopia. There may be tenderness and nodules over the distribution of the temporal arteries. The erythrocyte sedimentation rate is usually markedly elevated. This headache requires immediate treatment to prevent blindness.

PLAN:

Neurology consultation

All patients with persistent headaches or suspected intracranial lesions should be referred to a neurologist. The urgency will depend on the suspected disease.

Diagnostic
EEG
Brain scan

Useful screening procedures to rule out an intracranial lesion.

Therapeutic

Treatment is first directed to the underlying cause of the headache. For example, the patient with tension headache should have an exploration of the reasons underlying his problem. Hypertension should be controlled if present. Problems such as dental caries, sinusitis, mastoiditis should also be looked for and treated.

Other types of headaches can be treated with specific medications. The group of vascular headaches including common migraine, classic migraine and cluster headaches can be treated with ergotamine preparations. These must be given at onset of the headache or shortly after to be effective. They can be used prophylactically at bedtime for cluster headaches. Inciting causes for these headaches, such as emotional problems, birth control pills, should be looked for and removed. Long-term treatment for persistent problems in this area will require neurologic consultation and a more involved treatment regimen.

Temporal arteritis requires immediate steroid therapy and possibly hospitalization for further evaluation. Patients with suspected bacterial meningitis and subarachnoid hemorrhage also require immediate hospitalization.

In addition to the above specific treatments, there is also available a wide variety of analgesic medications. In general, one should start with the more simple remedies, such as aspirin and acetaminophen, possibly combined with propoxyphene before proceeding to the more potent analgesics. Antiemetics may be helpful in some cases. You should attempt to avoid narcotic analgesics, as the patient may become dependent on them, or evaluation of mental status may be obscured.

Patient education

This is extremely important. Headaches can be a persistent and debilitating problem. If no easily reversible cause is found, the patient should be instructed that his problem may require repeated visits, several evaluations and tests and some time before complete relief is afforded. The patient should be assured that you (or another nurse or a doctor) will work with him. If you feel a specific referral is needed (e.g. Neurology, Psychiatry), the reason for this should be explained.

Finally, the choice of medicines, the reasons for tests ordered and the need for follow-up should be discussed in some detail. The patient should be instructed to return sooner if his symptoms worsen or do not respond to the treatment regimen chosen.

BIBLIOGRAPHY

Lance, J. W.: *The Mechanisms and Management of Headache*, 2nd ed., Butterworth and Co., Ltd., London, 1973.

Wintrobe, M. W. et al. (eds.): *Harrison's Principles of Internal Medicine*, 8th ed., New York, McGraw-Hill, 1974.

Wolff, Harold George: *Headache and Other Head Pain*, 3rd ed., Oxford University Press, New York, 1972.

NOTES

Chapter 10

Low
back
pain

LOW BACK PAIN WORKSHEET

> To be used in patients with:
> Low Back Pain
> Back Problems
> Pain in Hip

> *What you can't afford to miss: aortic aneurysm, disc disease with paralysis, renal calculi (in patient with 1 kidney), sepsis.*

Chief Complaint:_____

SUBJECTIVE DATA:

DESCRIBE ALL POSITIVE RESPONSES
(Include Onset, Severity, Duration, Location)

Location: _____

Onset: _____

Duration: _____

Character: _____

Radiation: _____

Frequency: _____

Course: _____

Severity at worst: _____

Yes *No*

_____ _____ History of trauma: _____

_____

INVOLVES:
Yes *No*

_____ _____ Legal assistance _____

_____ _____ Workman's compensation: _____

_____ _____ Disability payment: _____

PRECIPITATING/AGGRAVATING FACTORS:
Yes *No*

_____ _____ Activity (work, occupation, position, exercises,

riding/driving): _____

_____ _____ Straining at stool: _____

_____ _____ After inactivity: _____

RELIEVED BY:
Yes *No*

_____ _____ Rest: _____

_____ _____ Position: _____

—— —— Therapy (check):

—————Medication:_____

—————Heat

—————Massage

—————Brace

—————Firm mattress

NOTE: If pain appears unrelated to trauma or activity, consider referred pain as etiology. See appropriate worksheet: Dysuria, Vaginal Discharge, Abdominal Pain, Chest Pain.

ASSOCIATED SYMPTOMS:

Yes   No

—— —— Numbness in extremities:_____

—— —— Tingling: _____

—— —— Weakness: _____

—— —— Atrophy: _____

—— —— Loss of sphincter control:

　　　　　Bowel: _____

　　　　　Bladder: _____

—— —— Paralysis:_____

—— —— Limitation of movement: _____

—— —— Stiffness: _____

—— —— Other joint pain: _____

—— —— Fever/chills: _____

___ ___ Night sweats: _____

___ ___ Weight loss: _____

___ ___ Fatigue: _____

PAST MEDICAL HISTORY:
Yes   No

___ ___ History of same back pain/previous back injury:

　　　　Diagnosis: _____

___ ___ Previous therapy:

　　　　Type: _____

　　　　Duration: _____

　　　　Outcome: _____

___ ___ Back surgery:

　　　　Type: _____

　　　　Date: _____

___ ___ Previous back x-rays:

　　　　Result: _____

　　　　Date: _____

___ ___ Other illnesses: _____

___ ___ Previous hospitalizations: _____

___ ___ Other surgery: _____

___ ___ Current medications: _____

_____

OBJECTIVE DATA:

DESCRIBE ALL POSITIVE RESPONSES

Vital signs: _____B/P _____P _____T _____Wt

General appearance: _____

Yes   *No*

—   —   Abnormal gait: _____

—   —   Uneven posture: _____

—   —   Unable to walk on toes:_____

—   —   Unable to walk on heels: _____

—   —   Decreased spinal mobility: _____

—   —   Pain with lateral bending: _____

—   —   Pain with hyperextension: _____

—   —   Pain with squatting: _____

—   —   Absent/unequal deep tendon reflexes:_____

—   —   Unequal leg length:

      Right:_____

      Left:_____

—   —   Abnormal sensation: _____

—   —   Decreased motor strength:

      _____Flexion-extension knee

      _____Dorsiflexion of great toe and foot

      _____Plantar flexion of ankle

___ ___ Positive straight leg raising (degrees):

Right:_____

Left:_____
(confirm by lowering leg and dorsiflexing ankle)

___ ___ Pain with hip rotation:

_____Internal: Right:_____ Left_____

_____External: Right_____ Left_____

___ ___ Spinal tenderness: _____

___ ___ Spinal deformity palpable: _____

LAB DATA:
*Done Not
     Done*

___ ___ Lumbosacral spine x-ray: _____

_____AP–lateral: _____

_____Obliques:_____

___ ___ CBC: _____

___ ___ Urinalysis: _____

___ ___ Erythrocyte sedimentation rate (ESR): _____

ASSESSMENT:

_____

_____

_____

_____

PLAN:

_____ Admit

_____ Consult:

    _____Orthopedics

    _____Neurosurgery

DIAGNOSTIC:

    _____Lumbosacral spine x-ray: _____

    _____AP–lateral

    _____Obliques

    _____Urine culture

    _____CBC

    _____ESR

    _____Rheumatoid factor

    _____Alkaline/acid phosphatase

    _____Protein electrophoresis

    _____Calcium

    _____Tine/PPD

THERAPEUTIC:

    _____Analgesia: _____

    _____Muscle relaxant: _____

    _____Antibiotic: _____

_____Other: _____

PATIENT EDUCATION:

_____Bedrest: _____

_____Firm mattress/bed board: _____

_____Heat: _____

_____Activity modification: _____

_____Correct body mechanics: _____

_____Back exercises: _____

_____Return appointment, especially if no improve-

ment/worsening: _____

_____

_____Referral to other clinic: _____

LOW BACK PAIN WORKSHEET RATIONALE

SUBJECTIVE DATA:

Location — Helps to determine if pain is local, referred or radicular. Local pain is rather diffuse but is always felt in or near the affected area of spine.

Onset — Sudden onset implies a specific event such as aneurysm rupture, strain while lifting. Gradual onset implies a more insidious process such as infection or tumor. What the patient was doing at the time of onset may also be a clue to etiology.

Duration — Short duration implies an acute process (e.g. disc, infection and tumor), although all chronic problems must start sometime. Duration of months to years implies a relatively benign process, (e.g. musculoskeletal), although ultimately the patient may be psychologically or physically crippled.

Character

Local: steady or intermittent ache

Referred: a. deep ache
b. retains characteristics of pain from affected organ

Radicular: intense, sharp

Radiation

Local: nonradiating

Referred: a. projected from spine into regions lying within area of lumbar and upper sacral dermatomes
b. projected from pelvic and abdominal viscera to the spine

Radicular: radiates from central spine to posterior aspect of the lower extremity

Frequency
Course

Musculoskeletal pain is typically intermittent and recurrent. Although a given episode may last several days, recurrences over the ensuing months or years are common. Frequency is related to the underlying process. Destructive diseases (tumor, infection) have a progressive course if untreated. Arthritis of varying types may cause intermittent pain with gradual destruction and deformity of the spine.

Severity at worst

This is not necessarily related to the severity of the underlying problem. Musculoskeletal pain or the pain of a ruptured disc may be severe, while the pain of tumor or infection may begin as a dull ache. Pain out of proportion to the objective findings may provide an insight into the patient's reaction to his problem.

History of trauma

A frequent cause of back pain, or point of reference for patient.

Legal assistance
  Workman's compensation
  Disability

Indicates need for more careful documentation and referral to the appropriate specialist (be alert to the patient who is "doctor-shopping" for best answer).

Aggravating Factors
  Activity

Frequent cause and aggravating factor since movement irritates sensory endings in traumatized musculoskeletal tissues.

  Straining at stool

Leads to increased radicular pain. Valsalva maneuver leads to increased intraspinal pressure which causes shift in position of root.

  After inactivity

Consider inflammatory arthritis.

Relieving Factors

True musculoskeletal back pain decreases with rest and symptomatic measures. This information is necessary to avoid unsuccessful modalities and determine patient compliance.

Associated Symptoms

Numbness in extremity	Indicates nerve root compression with hyposensitivity in dermatome pattern.
Tingling	As above, except with hypersensitivity.
Weakness	Indicates compression of motor root.
Atrophy	Indicates sustained motor nerve root compression.
Loss of sphincter control Paralysis	May occur with massive derangement of disc with nerve or cord damage.
Limitation of movement	May be due to muscle spasm, stiffness, pain or weakness.
Stiffness	Occurs with arthritis, muscle overuse and spasm.
Other joint pain	May indicate arthritis, other joint or connective tissue disorder.
Fever/chills	Rule out infection either local or systemic.
Night sweats	Rule out tuberculosis.
Weight loss	Rule out cancer.
Fatigue	Rule out cancer, systemic illness. This is a nonspecific symptom.

Past Medical History

History of similar pain	May give clue to diagnosis of present problem, particularly if symptoms are similar.

Previous therapy	This may show what has helped in the past. Also the extent, types and success of previous therapy gives an insight into how the patient copes with the illness.
Back surgery	This occasionally may aggravate as well as relieve pain. Surgery also implies documented nerve root or cord compression.
Previous back x-rays	These should be sent for and compared to the current set.
Other illnesses/ hospitalizations/surgery	This will give an indication of the patient's overall health in the past.
Current medications	In addition to any medicines for the back pain, it is important to know what other medicines the patient is taking to avoid drug interactions or additive effects.

OBJECTIVE DATA:

Vital signs Weight	These are generally taken to document the patient's present status. They should be normal with musculoskeletal back pain. Increased pulse and low blood pressure may be found with blood loss (e.g. leaking aneurysm) and demand immediate investigation.
General appearance	Watch for limitation of movement as patient walks into room, dresses, undresses, moves about. A great deal can be learned observing the patient when he is not overly self-conscious about being scrutinized.

Gait	Watch patient walk down hall, observing type of gait. A normal gait implies no serious nerve compression.
Posture	Note level of shoulders, pelvis, uneven carriage due to shorter extremity, scoliosis, "sciatic list," kyphosis, lordosis.
Unable to walk on toes	S-1 root; motor weakness of gastrocnemius.
Unable to walk on heels	L-5 root; motor weakness of the tibialis anticus.
Mobility of spine	*Flexion:* With disc disease, muscle spasm prevents motion and causes reversal or flattening of lumbar lordotic curve.
	Lateral bending: With a strain, bending away from affected side increases pain; with a disc causing nerve compression, bending toward the affected side increases pain.
	Hyperextension: Pressure on the vertebral bodies caused by hyperextension will increase pain of any inflammatory disease around the bodies. Strains are not usually affected and disc problems are affected only in their early phase.
Squatting	Produces flexion of knees and hips and can help localize pain in these areas.
Reflexes	L-5 root involvement: Ankle jerks are seldom diminished.

S-1—ankle jerk is diminished to absent in the majority of cases.

L-4, L-3—knee jerk is diminished or abolished.

Leg length

Unequal leg lengths alter line of weight bearing with resulting strain on muscles supporting the spine.

Sensation

Abnormalities are according to dermatomes affected (see p. 234—sensory dysfunction).

Motor strength

Evaluate muscle tone and mass.
Flexion and extension of knee—L-3 nerve root.
Dorsiflexion of great toe and foot—L-5 nerve root.
Plantar flexion of ankle—S-1 nerve root.

Straight leg raising

Is positive in acute and subacute attacks of lumbar disc lesions. Motion stretches nerve and causes nerve root irritation with pain in the back and/or sciatic distribution.

If test appears positive, you can confirm by lowering leg and dorsiflexing foot.

Pain produced by ligament or muscle pull is ruled out since dorsiflexion of the ankles will stretch the sciatic nerve.

Hip rotation

To rule out hip disease: pain with internal rotation indicates stress of the sacroiliac joint.

Pain with external rotation indicates hip disease.

Spinal tenderness/deformity

Palpate for tenderness and deformity. Percussion sensitivity is characteristic of Pott's disease, osteomyelitis or neoplasm. Hypersensitivity on palpation of transverse processes as well as overlying sacrospinal muscles may signify fracture of transverse process or strain of muscle attachments. Tenderness in the region of the articular facets between L-5 and S-1 is consistent with lumbar disc disease; it may also be due to rheumatoid arthritis. Any deviation of the spinous process in the anteroposterior or lateral direction may indicate spondylolisthesis.

Lab Data

AP–Lateral lumbosacral spine x-ray
Obliques

May indicate an abnormality.

Disc disease—may show no abnormality or at most a narrowing of the intervertebral space, sometimes more on the side of the rupture. May see "traction spur," fracture and congenital anomalies. Useful in spondylolisthesis where you may see forward displacement of vertebral body or "puppy-dog collar" defect. Degenerative changes such as osteophytic overgrowth, spur formation and ridging may be evident.

There is a straightening of the lordotic curve with muscle spasm.

Osteoporosis: May see collapsed vertebrae, wedging, decreased mineral density, "codfish vertebrae."

Destructive disease: First x-rays may not disclose lesions (nearly 1 cc. of bone must be destroyed in vertebral body before visible on x-ray).

Ankylosing spondylitis: Straightening of lumbar curve, squaring of lumbar and lower thoracic vertebrae.

Multiple myeloma: Punched-out bony lesions

CBC

Rule out infection, inflammation, anemia.

Urinalysis

To rule out urinary tract infection.

ESR

Nonspecific indicator of disease, increased in infections, inflammations, some neoplastic and collagen diseases.

ASSESSMENT:

Portions of the lower spine and pelvis, with their numerous muscular and tendinous attachments, are relatively inaccessible to palpation and also to inspection even through x-ray. With this lack of reliable physical signs and laboratory tests, it is often necessary to depend on the patient's history and behavior during the examination. Relying on the patient's description of the character, location and conditions which modify the pain should help in identifying the origin of the pain.

Back pain generally consists of three types: 1) local, 2) referred, 3) radicular.

LOCAL PAIN:

Caused by any pathologic process which impinges upon or irritates sensory endings. The most richly innervated are: periosteum, ligaments, muscles, synovial membranes, annulus fibrosis.

Specific causes of local pain are:

1. Trauma

    a. fracture
    b. strain

2. Congenital anomaly
    Spondylolisthesis

3. Faulty body mechanics

    a. unequal leg lengths
    b. scoliosis, kyphosis, lordosis
    c. disproportionate obesity

4. Arthritis

    a. osteoarthritis
    b. rheumatoid arthritis
    c. ankylosing spondylitis

5. Destructive diseases

    a. Infections

        1. tuberculosis
        2. acute hematogenous osteomyelitis

    b. Neoplastic

        1. primary sarcoma
        2. metastatic carcinoma

3. multiple myeloma

c. Metabolic

osteoporosis

Trauma

Fracture is usually the result of a flexion injury, as with a fall from heights; occasionally secondary to osteoporosis. The irritation of periosteum, stretching of ligaments, pressure from edema and hemorrhage, spasm, displacement of bone fragments causes pressure on meninges, pain and limitation of movement.

Sprain/strain: Due to incomplete tearing or stretching of the tendons and ligaments at the site of their attachment. Unusual use of muscles such as performing heavy work, especially lifting, pushing or pulling in a stooped position, sports, accidents, causes soreness and spasm.

It may be mild and persistent as a result of abnormal posture, since the strained tissues have to compensate for postural defects.

Congenital anomaly

Spondylolisthesis: The displacement of a portion of the spine onto the remainder; often lumbar. Displacement causes strain on adjacent ligaments and articulations resulting in protective muscle spasm.

Faulty body mechanics

Unequal leg lengths, dorsal kyphosis, increased lumbar lordosis, scoliosis: Alter the line of weight-bearing with a compensa-

tory strain of the muscles supporting the vertebral column.

Disproportionate obesity or pregnancy with forward displacement
and ptosis of the abdominal viscera
causes strain on the suspensory ligaments that attach to the back.

Arthritis

Osteoarthritis occurs in later life
with pain centered in the spine. It is
affected by position and associated
with stiffness and limitation of motion.

Rheumatoid arthritis may involve
the spine with associated active
inflammation of other joints with
pain, stiffness, limitation of motion.

Ankylosing spondylitis begins in
sacroiliac joint. Recurrent pain may
radiate, ascending dorsally. Aching
or stiffness present upon awaking in
morning and after inactivity. Not
particularly aggravated by physical
activity or movement. Occurs pre-
dominantly in males (5 to 1) and in
25-35 age group.

Destructive diseases

These are painless as long as limited to osseous tissue. With spread
to periosteum or adjacent spinous
structures they become the source
of local and referred pain.

Tuberculosis may affect one sacroiliac joint or vertebral column with
tenderness over affected area.

Pyogenic osteomyelitis may occur
spontaneously or may follow skin

infection, extension from adjacent infection, or urinary tract infection. Severe pain, low-grade fever. Both tuberculosis and pyogenic arthritis characteristically show nocturnal pain, spinal ache and percussion sensitivity.

Neoplastic, either primary or metastatic: Unrelenting, constantly progressive pain often in a patient with previous diagnosis of malignancy, who has insidious onset of low back pain.

Multiple myeloma: "Boring" pain, constant, increased with weight-bearing, movement; frequently presents with a fracture. Associated with a normocytic anemia.

Osteoporosis

Aching in lumbar or thoracic region. When marked, vertebrae may mold under the expansile pressure of the disc and produce strain on regional tissue. Minor injury may cause compression fracture.

REFERRED PAIN:

Is of 2 types: 1) pain projected from spine into regions lying within the area of the lumbar and upper sacral dermatomes, 2) pain projected from the pelvic and abdominal viscera to the spine.

Pain in the upper part of the lumbar spine is usually referred to the anterior aspects of the thighs and legs; that from the lower spine is referred to the gluteal regions, posterior thighs and calves. Maneuvers which alter local pain have a similar effect on referred pain.

The pain of diseases of the pelvic, abdominal or thoracic viscera is often felt in the region of the spine; i.e. it is referred to the more posterior parts of the spinal segment which innervates the diseased organ. Occasionally back pain may be the first positive sign.

Site of Pain	*Referred From*
a. Thoracic	a. Posterior parietal pleura
b. Lower thoracic, T-8 ⟶ L-2	b. Upper abdominal disease
c. Lumbar, L-2 → L-4	c. Lower abdominal disease
d. Sacral	d. Pelvis
e. Thoracic, lumbar	e. Aneurysm
f. Costovertebral angle	f. Kidney
g. Lumbar ⟶ low abdomen ⟶ genitals	g. Ureter, renal stone

Characteristically, there are no local signs; e.g. no stiffness of the back. Range of motion is full without augmentation of the pain. The pain retains the characteristics (e.g. onset, duration) of pain from the affected organ.

RADICULAR OR ROOT PAIN:

Has some of the characteristics of referred pain but differs in its greater intensity, distal radiation, circumscription to the territory of a nerve root, and in the factors that excite it. The mechanism is distention, stretching, irritation or compression of a spinal root, most often central to the intervertebral foramen. The pain is sharp, intense, nearly always radiates from the spine to some lower extremity.

Fully developed syndrome of ruptured intervertebral disc includes backache, abnormal posture and limitation of motion.

Nerve root involvement is also indicated by sensory disturbances and motor abnormalities. Most likely to occur between L-5 and S-1, with lessening frequency between L-4, L-5; L-3, L-4; L-2, L-1. Cause is usually a flexion injury, and in many cases no trauma is recalled. Degeneration of the posterior longitudinal ligaments and annulus fibrosis, which occurs in most adults of middle and advanced years, may have taken place silently or been manifested by a mild recurrent lumbar ache. A sneeze, lurch or other trivial movement may then precipitate disc protrusion.

Location of pain:

Compression of L-5 roots: low back and/or hip within posterolateral thigh ⟶ calf ⟶ lateral aspects ankle ⟶ occasionally dorsal aspect foot ⟶ 1st, 2nd, 3rd toes.

Compression of S-1 roots: low back and/or hip ⟶ posterolateral thigh ⟶ calf ⟶ heel ⟶ plantar surface of foot ⟶ 4th, 5th toes.

Compression of L-3, L-4 roots: anterior thigh and knee.

Area of sensory dysfunction (numbness, tingling)	Sensory disturbances are hyper-, hyposensitivity in a dermatome pattern.

Compression of L-5 roots: paresthesia may be in entire territory, or only in distal parts (see above location).

S-1 roots: mainly in lower leg, outer toes.

L-3, L-4: anterior thigh and knee. |
| Area of motor dysfunction (weakness, atrophy) | Motor abnormalities are usually less prominent than pain and sensory symptoms and signs.

Compression of L-5 roots: weakness, if present, involves extensors of big toe and of the foot.

S-1 roots: flexor muscles of the foot and toes, abductors of the toe, hamstring muscles.

L-3, L-4: quadriceps weakness. |

PLAN:

Diagnostic

Orthopedic/neurosurgery consult	Should be done if there are objective sensory or motor abnormalities. Immediate consultation is mandatory if there is bladder or bowel dysfunction.
X-rays	See Lab Data section.
Urine culture	Do if urinalysis suggests infection.
CBC ESR	See Lab Data section.

Rheumatoid factor	To help rule out rheumatoid arthritis.
Alkaline/acid phosphatase	To help rule out malignancy. Most of these enzymes in the body are produced by bone, and with disease and increased osteoblastic activity, the levels increase.
Protein electrophoresis	To rule out multiple myeloma with the presence of myeloma protein.
Calcium	This may increase to toxic levels in malignant diseases involving bone.
Tine/PPD	To help diagnose tuberculosis.

Therapeutic
Analgesia	Individualize choice of drug and dosage. Be liberal first few days. Strong analgesics (e.g. narcotics) may be necessary with disc disease.
Muscle relaxant	May be helpful although their effectiveness has not been documented.
Antibiotic	For urinary tract infections.

Patient education
Bedrest	Immobilization in a recumbent position that relaxes and removes pressure from the injured structure. This is the cornerstone of treatment, and 7-10 days of complete bedrest may be necessary.
Firm mattress/bed board	
Heat	Improves circulation. Relaxes spasm.
Activity modification	Avoidance of activity that favors spinal injury, e.g. heavy lifting.

Correct body mechanics	To avoid strain, injury. Instruct patient on how to lift objects with back straight and on necessity of correct posturing.
Back exercises	To strengthen trunk muscles, overcome faulty position and increase mobility of spinal joints.
Return appointment or return if worsening, no improvement	Patient should expect muscle strain to take 2-4 weeks to improve. Ligamentous strain: 6-12 weeks. Acute disc: 2-3 weeks.
Referral to other clinic/specialist	*Orthopedic/neurosurgery:* If symptoms don't resolve or if objective sensory or motor abnormalities develop.

BIBLIOGRAPHY

Finneson, Bernard E.: *Low Back Pain,* Philadelphia: Lippincott, 1972.

Gibbens, Murray E.: "Diagnosis and Treatment of Low Back Pain," *American Journal of Orthopedic Surgery,* pp. 218–221, August-September 1968.

Riordan, Forrest H., III and Donald H. Holder: "The Painful Back," *Hospital Medicine,* pp. 33–47, June 1973.

MacBryde, C. M. (ed.): *Signs and Symptoms,* 5th ed., Philadelphia: Lippincott, 1970.

Wintrobe, M. W. et al.: *Harrison's Principles of Internal Medicine,* 7th ed., New York: McGraw Hill, 1974.

Chapter 11

Rash–skin problems

RASH–SKIN PROBLEMS WORKSHEET

To be used in patients with:
Rash
Sores
Hives
Itching
Skin Problems

What you can't afford to miss: secondary syphilis, gonococcemia.

Chief Complaint:_____
SUBJECTIVE DATA:

Onset: _____Sudden _____Gradual _____Date commenced

Duration: _____

Location–distribution: _____

Character (describe): _____

Course: _____Constant _____Progressive

_____Intermittent _____Subsiding

Frequency–recurrences: _____

DESCRIBE POSITIVE RESPONSES
(Include Onset, Severity, Duration)

RELATED TO:
Yes　*No*

____　____　Occupation: _____

____　____　Leisure activities: _____

____　____　Foods: _____

____　____　Drug ingestion: _____

____　____　Physical factors (heat, cold, sunlight): _____

____　____　Season: _____

____　____　Environment (plants, chemicals, animals, cosmetics): ____

_____

____　____　Geographical factors: _____

ASSOCIATED SYMPTOMS:
Yes　*No*

____　____　Pruritus: _____

____　____　Pain: _____

____　____　Paresthesia: _____

____　____　Fever/chills: _____

____　____　Respiratory infection: _____

____　____　Other systemic symptoms (weight loss, malaise): _____

_____

____ ____ Current or previous treatment for above: _____

_____

_____

PAST MEDICAL HISTORY (include past and current medical and surgical problems):

_____

_____

_____

____ ____ Other medications: _____

____ ____ Allergies: _____

SEXUAL HISTORY:

_____

_____

_____

_____

FAMILY HISTORY:

_____

_____

_____

_____

Patient's opinion of cause: _____

_____

DESCRIBE POSITIVE FINDINGS

OBJECTIVE DATA:
General appearance: _____

SKIN EXAM: _____Not Done

_____

_____

_____

HAIR/SCALP EXAM: _____Not Done

_____

_____

_____

MOUTH AND PHARYNX EXAM: _____Not Done

_____

_____

_____

NAIL EXAM: _____Not Done

_____

_____

_____

LYMPH NODE EXAM: _____Not Done

_____

_____

_____

SPLEEN EXAM: _____Not Done

_____

_____

GENITAL EXAM: _____Not Done

_____

_____

OTHER EXAM: _____Not Done

_____

_____

_____

LAB DATA:
Done Not
       Done

____ ____ CBC with differential: ___WBC ___HCT ___HGB

Differential: _____

_____

____ ____ ESR: _____

____ ____ VDRL: _____

____ ____ KOH preparation:_____

____ ____ Gram stain:_____

____ ____ Culture:

_____Bacterial: _____

_____Fungal:_____

_____Viral: _____

___ ___ Darkfield: _____

___ ___ Tzanck smear: _____

___ ___ Cellophane tape: _____

___ ___ Diascopy:_____

___ ___ Wood's light: _____

ASSESSMENT:

_____

_____

_____

_____

PLAN:

_____ Admit to hospital: _____

_____ Referral: _____

THERAPEUTIC: _____

_____

_____

_____

DIAGNOSTIC: _____

_____

_____

_____

PATIENT EDUCATION: _____

_____

_____

_____

RASH-SKIN PROBLEM WORKSHEET RATIONALE

SUBJECTIVE DATA:

Onset	All should be determined as accu-
Duration	rately as possible in order to
Location/distribution*	give a logical picture of the de-
Character	velopment of the disease. Describe
Course	the original lesions and any sub-
Frequency	sequent change in appearance or
	character that the patient may have
	noted. Include the rate of enlarge-
	ment of lesions and the pattern of
	extension. Include dates of exacer-
	bations and recurrences.

Related to: Since the skin is the interface between man and his environment,
the patient must be questioned in
detail about the substances with
which he comes in contact, to determine the possible etiology of
skin problems.

Occupation — Ask about prolonged exposure to
Leisure activities — sunlight, carcinogens, chemicals, irritants.

Foods — Consider the ingestion of new
foods. Shellfish and fruit are sometimes responsible for skin eruptions.

*See Table 11-1, p. 271

Drug ingestion

Inquire about prescription medicines, any injections by doctors or dentists, and the use of over-the-counter medicines including cold remedies, laxatives, linaments, douches, eye and ear preparations, tonics, headache preparations.

Physical factors

The possibility of photosensitivity reactions or recurrences with exposure to heat or cold should be investigated.

Season

Time of appearance can be important. The patient with atopic dermatitis often worsens in winter; the sudden onset in spring of contact dermatitis might be due to poison ivy. It is important to consider the relationship between sun exposure and photodermatitis.

Environment

The patient may be sensitive to plants, chemicals or animals in his environment. Inquire about living conditions, economic and nutritional status. This will also help in determining treatment that is realistic and practical.

Geographical factors

Ask about past and present places of residence and travel. Both are associated with an increase in the risk of significant exposures to environmental agents.

Associated Symptoms:
Pruritus

Itching is a form of pain but, curiously, is itself often relieved by inducing local pain through scratching.

The responsible nerve fibers arise in the epidermis. The signals for itching are transmitted by chemical mediators including histamine and kallikrein, which are released by injury to the epidermis.

Onset of itching can be sudden, severe and generalized, or mild and well localized. The patient with pruritus may or may not present with an obvious pruritic lesion.

Pain
Paresthesia

Common with herpetic infections, especially herpes zoster in the older patient.

Fever/chills

Seen in serum sickness usually 7-10 days after the implicated exposure and is associated with joint pain. Seen in infectious diseases, including gonococcemia.

Respiratory infection

Symptoms of upper respiratory infection often precede or accompany viral exanthems.

Other systemic symptoms

Some skin disorders chiefly involve the skin while others are manifestations of an internal disorder.

Current or previous treatment

Self-treatment of skin lesions is extremely common, and the underlying condition may be concealed or replaced by the effects of inappropriate treatment.

Past Medical History:

Past illnesses and treatments may give insight into the present problem. Many skin problems have their root in systemic illnesses and/or medications. If the etiology of the rash is unclear, a detailed investigation of the past history is mandatory.

Sexual History: Should cover the patient's pattern of sexual activity including sexual preferences, since both gonorrhea and syphilis are more common in homosexuals. Ask about past history of venereal disease and current symptomatology of gonorrhea or syphilis in patient or sexual partner. This includes dysuria, urethral or vaginal discharge, abdominal pain, genital or oral lesion.

Family History: Helpful chiefly if history of atopic disorders is present. Ask about childhood asthma, hay fever and/or childhood atopic dermatitis (eczema) in family members.

Patient's Opinion of Cause: Should always be asked since it may be correct; if not, patient's fears about the possible cause of the problem can be dealt with specifically.

OBJECTIVE DATA:

General appearance The patient should be fully disrobed. Light must be adequate, and natural daylight is preferred for examination. Describe the patient, his mental status and his hygiene.

Skin Exam After inspection and palpation, lesions are described according to anatomic distribution, the configuration of groups of lesions and the morphology of individual lesions (see Table 11-1).

Hair/Scalp Exam	Evidence of pediculosis, seborrhea; alopecia seen in syphilis may be found.
Mouth and Pharynx Exam	Look for syphilitic chancre, for signs of viral/bacterial infections including vesicles, petechiae, exudate, Koplik's spots, tonsillitis.
Nail Exam	Pitting of nails is seen in psoriasis. The nail is chalky white at its free edge and friable and fragmented in fungal infections.
Lymph Node Exam	May find tender regional adenopathy with syphilis and with viral/bacterial infections.
Spleen Exam	The spleen may be enlarged with some viral illnesses (e.g. mononucleosis and occasionally hepatitis).
Genital Exam	Evidence of syphilitic chancre, fungal infections, herpes simplex may be found.

Lab Data:

CBC with differential	To evaluate the presence of infections. Leukocytosis occurs with bacterial infection; leukopenia and lymphocytosis with viral infection; eosinophilia is seen with allergies and certain parasites.
ESR	General indicator of inflammation.
VDRL	The serologic test for syphilis. Rarely becomes positive until 1 week after appearance of the chancre and sometimes not for 6 weeks.

KOH preparation
(10–40 % potassium
hydroxide)

To determine presence of fungus or yeast. *Procedure:* apply KOH to single small portion of scales on slide; top with coverslip and heat gently. Look for branching, segmented hyphae and/or spores.

Gram stain

For detection of microorganisms, chiefly bacteria and Candida.

Culture

To detect bacteria, virus, or fungus.

Darkfield

To detect *Treponema pallidum* of syphilis. Serum from erosions on male and female genitalia is examined. Test is not helpful with oral lesions because of the presence of nonpathogenic treponemas which are indistinguishable from the *Treponema pallidum.*

Tzanck smear

To detect giant multinucleate cells in herpes zoster, varicella and herpes simplex. *Procedure:* Material from base of vesicle is gently curetted and spread on glass slide. It is then stained with Wright-Giemsa stain and viewed under oil immersion.

Cellophane tape

To detect organism causing tinea versicolor. Apply tape to lesion, then attach to slide and look for hyphae and spores.

Diascopy

Used to differentiate purpura from erythematous macules. A glass slide is pressed over the lesion; purpura does not blanch while telangiectasias and some hemangiomas do.

Wood's light	Used to detect tinea capitis through yellow fluorescence of involved area; tinea versicolor imparts a white or pale yellow fluorescence. Observe suspected lesion or area in darkened room with ultraviolet light.

ASSESSMENT AND PLAN:

The etiology of rash and skin problems is often complex and interrelated with coexisting health problems. This section will cover the conditions which are potentially hazardous if missed on first encounter, and some of the more common conditions seen in practice.

I. Conditions Which You Can't Afford To Miss:

Gonococcemia	1-3 % of persons with gonorrhea develop gonococcemia. Both males and females may be asymptomatic until the septicemia develops, or they may have had symptoms such as dysuria, urethral or vaginal discharge and abdominal pain. History of intercourse with new or multiple partners is significant. If the organism has been dormant, the signs of systemic infection in females (in whom it is more common) may come with early pregnancy or soon after menstruation. The history may include rash, fever, malaise, polyarthralgias, arthritis and tenosynovitis, especially of wrists and Achilles tendon.
	The typical lesion is first a small papule on an erythematous base, which becomes a vesicle and then a pustule, sometimes with a necrotic center. Usually, there are only a few lesions, 3-20, on the distal extremities.

Gram-negative intracellular diplococci may be seen on a gram stain of scrapings from pustular lesions. The patient should usually be hospitalized for intravenous antibiotics, although the U.S. Public Health Service has stated that outpatient treatment is acceptable if there is no fluid in any joints and the patient is not severely ill.

Secondary syphilis

The patient may give a history of exposure to syphilis 2-6 months previous, followed by appearance of a single, painless, circular ulcer with firm margin and clear base on the genitalia or in mouth or lips.

The rash of secondary syphilis is a scaling maculopapular generalized eruption, including palms and soles, associated with enlarged, nontender regional lymph nodes. Sometimes fever, malaise, headache and generalized lymphadenopathy are present. Patchy scalp hair loss described as motheaten is sometimes seen. Annular lesions of the face occur, especially in blacks; flat warts of the genitalia, condylomata lata, also can be seen.

Lab diagnosis:

Lesion: darkfield visualization of spirochetes. *VDRL:* test for nonspecific antibodies. *Fluorescent Treponemal Antibody-Absorbed:* (FTA-ABS) Specific immunofluorescent treponemal antibody.

Biological false positive serology results can be caused by lupus erythematosus, pregnancy and use of heroin.

Treatment: 2.4 million units of benzathine penicillin G intramuscularly. Follow with serial VDRL's every 3 months for 1 year, then again at 2 years. Tetracycline and erythromycin are alternatives for treatment. Some patients have a temporary flare of cutaneous signs hours after treatment, called Herxheimer reaction.

II. Common Dermatologic Problems

Atopic dermatitis
(Generalized
neurodermatitis)

This problem is often chronic and recurring and can be lifelong. Hereditary, allergenic and psychogenic factors may be involved. The patient or close family members may have an atopic history—atopic dermatitis, hay fever and asthma. Atopic dermatitis sometimes begins as eczema in infancy. The process involves an antigen—antibody reaction in the epidermis and the mechanism involves increased immunoglobulin (IgE) levels. Pruritus is the chief complaint, and the skin changes seen are often secondary to scratching. Stress and sweat retention can aggravate the pruritus.

Subjective

Itching, rash.

Objective

A pruritic eruption of the face, neck, scalp, hands, wrists, popliteal and antecubital spaces is found. It is usually bilateral and symmetrical. Thickened, lichenified dry skin with papules and excoriations is seen. Secondary infection with crusting and oozing lesions can occur especially in children, but not before the age of 2 months.

Plan

Local steroids. Occlusive dressings should be avoided. Tranquilizers and antihistamines are useful.

Education

Use mild soaps and bath oil; avoid frequent drying baths, wool and other irritants. Avoid rapid changes in temperature, overheating and overexercise.

Small pox vaccination is contraindicated if the patient or family has active skin lesions, as eczema vaccinatum may result.

Contact dermatitis

One of the commonest skin problems. This is a reaction to irritants. It is a disease of specific immune origin where intercellular edema results in gross vesicles. The palms and soles have a low incidence of involvement because they are not easily penetrated by allergens. Contact allergens include: plants, drugs, cosmetics, metals, plastics, fabrics, dyes, handled foods, pollens, fungus spores.

Subjective

Rash, itching.

Objective

Lesions are circumscribed, red, weeping and vesiculobullous with swelling and scaling. The areas of the body involved with common specific allergies are:

Scalp: hats, hairnets
Ears: eyeglass frames, earrings

Face: eye and nose drops, lipstick, powder, cosmetics
Wrists and neck: jewelry, furs, clothing
Axilla: clothing, deodorants
Arms, legs, trunk: clothing, soaps
Arms, legs: plants
Feet: shoes and socks

Plan

Diagnosis by patch testing.
Avoidance of cause.
Burow's solution as cool compresses for 1 hour 4 times a day until resolution.
Topical steroids for inflammation.

Drug eruption

This can mimic many other dermatoses. A principle to remember is that a single drug can cause a different eruption in different people and that a given eruption can be caused by a variety of drugs.

Subjective

Rash, usually of sudden onset and bright red, often pruritic. Penicillin is the most common cause, though salicylates, barbiturates, bromides, iodides, sulfonamides, broad spectrum antibiotics and anticonvulsants can be implicated.

Objective

Small red macules, papules, vesicles or wheals, though one type of lesion predominates. Distribution is usually generalized and symmetrical.

Plan

Discontinue the offending drug.
Give antihistamines if necessary for itching. If bullae are present, aspirate them and apply warm wet soaks.

Avoid soap.

If reaction is severe, give oral steroids. The dosage is initially large, then tapered quickly over 5-10 days.

Erythema multiforme

This is a cutaneous hypersensitivity reaction with a variety of causes, including drugs such as sulfonamides, salicylates, bromides and penicillin, infection, vaccines, especially smallpox, herpes simplex and malignancy.

Subjective

Itching, lesions and sometimes malaise, fever in the bullous stage.

Objective

Sharply outlined, round, symmetrical, erythematous, maculopapular, bull's-eye lesions of various sizes, often associated with nodules, or bullae of skin and mucous membranes. The bullous form involving the skin and mucous membranes is called Stevens-Johnson syndrome.

Plan

Thorough investigation to determine cause. Short course of systemic steroids in less severe cases. In severe attacks, such as Stevens-Johnson syndrome, massive doses of steroids are often used.

With oral mucous membrane involvement, advise a liquid diet and antihistamine or viscous lidocaine mouthwash.

Fixed drug eruption

This reaction represents an island of hypersensitivity.

Subjective

Patients will give a history of a recurrent lesion at one or more spots.

Most often responsible are barbiturates and phenolphthalein, which is found in some toothpastes and laxatives. However, any drug (commonly tetracycline, sulfonamides, penicillin, aspirin, quinine or ephedrine), or chemical taken internally can be responsible.

Objective

There are a few large, oval, red or purple papules that recur in exactly the same spot when the causative agent is given and subside when it is withdrawn, leaving some residual hyperpigmentation. Wrists and ankles are often the site, and the lesions are asymmetrical.

Plan

Avoid the causative agent.

Herpes zoster

This is a viral infection believed due to the same virus that causes varicella. There are disseminated, multiorgan and encephalomyelitic forms. The assessment can be difficult to make during the prodrome, and occasionally no skin changes are ever present. Thus with the sudden onset of segmental pain, zoster should be considered.

The trigger to disease can be malignancy, radiation therapy, lumbar puncture, neurosurgery or immunosuppressive therapy, although usually no inciting event is found.

The varicella virus is thought to become caged in the dorsal root ganglia, and after its release to reproduce along one ganglionic pathway. It invades the corresponding dermatome and produces the characteristic skin changes. Postherpetic neuralgia is often seen.

Subjective

Persistent, burning, aching pain with segmental distribution. The thorax is a common site; the trigeminal and cervical nerves are often affected. Skin lesions are tender.

Objective

Bands of grouped vesicles with an erythematous base along peripheral nerves with corresponding enlarged tender lymph nodes. Tzanck smear of vesicular fluid reveals multinucleate giant cells as in varicella or herpes simplex. There may be adenitis of the regional lymph nodes.

Plan

Analgesia. 1% lidocaine block for temporary relief in the acute stage. Steroids can be used in severe cases and may help prevent postherpetic neuralgia.

Refer to ophthalmologist if eye involved, because of possible damage to cornea.

Try to determine the trigger, or if malignancy is present.

Herpes simplex

Herpes simplex is a cutaneous viral infection, though it can travel on the surface of the body and along nerves, resulting in meningoencephalitis. It is highly infectious, and patients with disease should avoid direct contact with the following: infants; patients with burns, eczema or abraded skin; patients with immunologic deficiencies related to leukemia; those receiving immunosuppressive therapy; or inheritance. The course is protracted with recurrence and sometimes complicated by secondary bacterial infection.

Subjective

Vesicular lesions are sometimes associated with constitutional signs (malaise, fever), and preceded by pain, tingling, burning.

Objective

Painful vesicular eruption with swelling, lymphangitis, lymphadenopathy and fever. The mucosa can be involved as well as tonsils, pharynx and the eye including the conjunctiva, cornea and other structures.

Diagnosis confirmed by presence of multinucleate giant cells on Tzanck smear; also by biopsy and culture.

Most nongenital herpes is due to herpes virus type I.

Most genital herpes is due to herpes virus type II. This type can be dangerous during pregnancy because of perinatal infection during delivery. It also is the most common cause of genital lesion in females and second only to syphilis in males.

Plan

Treatment with agents that interfere with viral replication is controversial. Health care personnel should be advised always to wear gloves when doing oral hygiene on patients.

Education

The process is self-limited; usually lasts about 10 days. Precipitants can be fever, sunburn, stress and menses.

Impetigo

This problem is more common in childhood. There is often a history of exposure to someone with impetigo or respiratory infection, or the patient may have had a preceding upper respiratory infection.

Subjective

Rash; lesions, usually of face, hands or other exposed surfaces.

Objective

Circular, vesiculopustular, crusting erosions are seen. There may be central drying which results in round lesions with central clearing and peripheral crusting. Cultures show coagulase-positive staphylococci or beta hemolytic streptococci.

Plan

Systemic antibiotics. Erythromycin is the 1st choice.

Education

Wash lesions carefully to remove crusts. Otherwise keep hands away from lesions and use frequent handwashing. The lesions will heal without scarring.

Impetigo with Group A beta hemolytic streptococci may precede acute glomerulonephritis.

Molluscum contagiosum

A viral disease found only in man and chimpanzees, characterized by the uniformity of the lesions which affect only the epidermis. The infection is more common in children, and is passed by autoinoculation with close contact.

Subjective	Usually asymptomatic.
Objective	Multiple, small, discrete, pale, pearly or miliary, firm papules with a central umbilication. A keratinous, cheese-like substance can be expressed from the center. Usually found on the face, arms and genitalia.
Plan	If there are only a limited number of lesions, one may prick with a needle to open lesion, curette, freeze and desiccate. However, they often resolve spontaneously.
	If diffuse, look for underlying cause such as immune deficit; treat lesions with topical vitamin A acid.
Nummular eczema	Adults with dry skin are affected more often than children. It is common during winter with the associated increased dryness, and is often gone by summer. It can recur at the same site and is aggravated by too frequent bathing.
Subjective	May be pruritic.
Objective	Circumscribed pink to red scaling, crusting, papulovesicular coin-shaped lesions. KOH is negative for fungi.
Plan	No soap and water. Coal tar; topical steroids with occlusive dressings.

Pediculosis

Pediculosis capitis.

Subjective

Pruritus of scalp.

Objective

Pear-shaped, transparent ova (nits) are usually seen on hair. Occasionally papulopustular lesions are seen. The louse, approximately 2 mm. long, can sometimes be found in crusted pustular lesions.

Pediculosis corporis: Like pediculosis capitis, this condition is often associated with poor hygiene.

Subjective

Pruritus of trunk and buttocks.

Objective

Linear excoriations are seen on the trunk with diffuse hyperpigmentation. The lice are slightly longer than in pediculosis capitis, and lice and nits are usually found in seams of clothing. Lice fluoresce white under Wood's light.

Pediculosis pubis: There may be a history of sexual contact with a new partner or a symptomatic partner.

Subjective

Pruritus of pubic area.

Objective

Adult parasites are easily seen. The 1.5 mm. brownish insects can be seen with the naked eye and magnification shows that two of the six legs have claws, thus the common term "crabs." Ova can be seen on the pubic hair shaft as well as the eyelashes. Blue-brown macules may be present on the skin.

Plan

Several applications of 1 % gamma benzene solution with retreatment

1 week later, if necessary. Disinfect bedclothes and clothing at time of treatment.

Perioral dermatitis

A condition that seems to be induced by the use of topical steroids, though it may be a variant of seborrheic dermatitis, or due to some changes in the oral flora. It is a disease of females, may persist for years, and appears only around the mouth. It is not associated with any internal disease.

Subjective

Rash and itching.

Objective

Pruritic erythematous papules and pustules around the chin and lips, often with a clear area adjacent to the vermilion border.

Plan

No topical steroids.
Tetracycline. Give before meals and not with iron, which decreases its absorption.

Pityriasis rosea

This skin problem is thought to be a viral exanthem or an autoimmune phenomenon. It affects young adults and the middle-aged. It lasts 6-8 weeks, resolves with no residual scarring, is not likely to recur, is not contagious and is not a sign of ill health.

Subjective

Rash on trunk. The face is not involved.

Objective

Multiple, small, oval or round, pink, macular lesions with scaling centers, or small papules with a central ring of scale. The long axis of the lesions is arranged parallel to the lines of cleavage of the skin. It is usually preceded days to weeks by a single, large, oval "herald patch."

Plan

Therapy is usually unnecessary, but steroid cream can be applied to the lesions. Excessive bathing and irritants should be avoided. Do VDRL to rule out secondary syphilis.

Psoriasis

The cause of psoriasis is unknown, but it is a chronic process that may be due to abnormal epidermal protein metabolism. It can often be related to some mechanical trauma to the skin, such as resting elbows on desks, fatigue or environmental changes.

Subjective

Onset is often in the 2nd decade of life and is usually asymptomatic.

Objective

The lesions are round, flat, translucent or silvery, barely elevated papules with some scaling; there may be dense white scales with underlying bleeding after the removal of scales. Lesions are sharply circumscribed. It can involve the scalp, buttock cleft, extensor surfaces, especially knees and elbows, or the entire skin. Involvement of nails is reflected in pitting of the nail plate or thick yellow nails.

Plan

Protect area involved from mechanical trauma. Topical steroid ointment or cream with plastic wrap–occlusive dressing.

Scabies

Caused by the *Sarcoptes scabiei* mite, and can occur in meticulously clean patients as well as those with poor hygiene. It does not occur on the face but is commonly seen in finger webs, wrists, skin folds and nails.

Subjective

Pruritus, characteristically worse at night.

Objective

Characteristic lesion is the burrow—a straight or twisted thread-like line seen under the skin where the mite has deposited its eggs. Excoriated papules and tiny vesicles are also seen.

Plan

Apply scabicide from the neck down and leave it on. Repeat in 24 hours. Take cleansing bath several hours after the second application. Change and disinfect clothing at time of cleansing bath. Check all contacts. The incubation period is 3 weeks.

Seborrheic dermatitis

Seborrheic dermatitis affects areas rich in sebaceous glands, is associated with oily scalp and skin and is sometimes seen in patients with acne. Tension may be associated with flare-ups, and secondary bacterial infection sometimes occurs. Need to consider sensitivity to hair products and presence of psoriasis with its thick, discrete plaques which may affect the scalp.

Subjective

Itching and scaling.

Objective

Pruritic diffuse (not patchy) scaling, greasy, red, crusted, symmetrical lesions affecting scalp, eyebrows, nasolabial area, postauricular, sternal, interscapular areas and eyelids.

Plan

Frequent use of antiseborrheal shampoos and topical preparations containing sulfur, tar and salicylic acid which debrides the keratin scaling.

Steroids or antibiotics may be necessary in extensive or severe cases.

A low-fat, low-carbohydrate, high-protein diet may or may not be helpful.

Stasis dermatitis

Underlying conditions include chronic venous insufficiency caused by venous obstruction, congestive heart failure, incompetency of deep venous valves, varicose veins or lymphatic obstruction.

Subjective

Itching, red, scaling and/or oozing lesions of lower legs.

Objective

Edema, erythema, fissures, scaling, oozing ulcers, increased pigmentation, purpura, petechiae of lower legs, especially the medial surface.

Plan

Topical preparations including zinc oxide.
Avoid soap and other drying agents.
Elastic bandages applied before getting out of bed.
Frequent rest in supine position with legs elevated 15°.
Surgical treatment includes ligation of incompetent perforating veins.

Tinea corporis

This is ringworm, an infectious skin problem whose source is fungi from animals, humans or soil. It may mimic other conditions including contact dermatitis, seborrhea and psoriasis.

Subjective

Itching; may be asymptomatic.

Objective

Expanding, annular, red-rimmed lesions with central scaling. Slightly elevated plaques, 0.5–1.0 cm. in diameter, with a sharp margin and crusting. Central healing may leave rings or areas of erythema and scaling on the face, trunk, neck and hands. Epidermal scrapings (KOH preparation) show fungal hyphae.

Plan

Cleansing of loose scales followed by application of tolnaftate in propylene glycol (Tinactin). If no response give griseofulvin by mouth.

Tinea versicolor

This is a noninflammatory fungal infection that follows the distribution of the sebaceous glands, except that the scalp is not affected. Its course is chronic and recurrences are frequent. Living in tropic regions, malnutrition and steroids all change skin flora and seem to predispose to this condition.

Subjective

Asymptomatic; usually presents as a cosmetic problem. Tanning accentuates the hypopigmented areas.

Objective

Noninflammatory tan, reddish-brown or white scaling patches that are round or irregular and found on the upper back, shoulders and neck. Lesions characteristically have a hyperpigmented scale and hypopigmented epidermis, with a fine, delicate, whitish, powdery scale.

The patches show yellowish fluorescence with Wood's light. KOH preparation of scales shows hyphae.

Plan

Bathing and vigorous rubbing to remove scales. 5 minute application of selenium sulfide shampoo to entire body, repeated daily until scales not apparent.

Verify cure by Wood's light.

Viral exanthems

A wide variety of cutaneous lesions are seen with viral infections, and their description will be dealt with according to causative viral agent.

Cytomegalovirus (CMV)

Is rarely associated with a red, maculopapular rash.

Infectious mononucleosis Epstein-Barr virus

Fever, malaise, pharyngitis, headache and abdominal pain.

Exudative pharyngitis and tonsillitis; lymphadenopathy characteristically including occipital adenopathy and splenomegaly.

Rash: 15 % have macular or maculopapular rash on trunk. This is more frequent in females than males by a ratio of 2:1.

CBC shows lymphocytosis or monocytosis with atypical lymphocytes. There is a positive heterophil, and frequently mild elevations of liver function tests.

Adenovirus

Symptoms of respiratory infection.

A wide variety of rashes is seen including macular, maculopapular, petechial.

Enterovirus

Fever, headache, coryza. Especially in summer and fall.

ECHO virus types 4 and 9 can cause a discrete maculopapular or petechial rash that is centrifugal and lasts 3–5 days.

Coxsackie

Hand, foot and mouth disease caused by types A16, 15, 10.

Fever, rash. Usually there is no coryza or cough.

90 % of patients with these types have a vesicular lesion on the oral mucosa and tongue. The body rash is maculopapular, becoming vesicular on digital portions of hands, feet including palms and soles.

Rubeola

Three day prodrome of fever, conjunctivitis, coryza, cough, photophobia and lassitude.

Koplik's spots, white specks on an erythematous base on buccal mucosa, are usually seen 1–2 days before onset of the generalized rash.

Rash is centrifugal and maculo-papular, and spreads from hairline and face over the body during a 3 day period. The CBC shows a leukopenia with lymphocytosis. Complications include otitis media, pneumonia, encephalitis.

Rubella

Little or no prodrome.

Macular or maculopapular discrete rash that starts on the face and ears, and spreads over body in about 3 days. Lymphadenopathy, primarily occipital and postauricular, begins 2–3 days before appearance of the rash.

The infection with the rash generally resolves spontaneously; there is no specific treatment.

PLAN:
Admit to hospital

Patients with severe systemic infection (e.g. gonococcemia) should be hospitalized. If a rash is widespread and requires intensive therapy, the patient usually can be more easily treated in the hospital. Viral infections with central nervous system involvement require inpatient observation.

Referral

Dermatology consult is needed in all diagnostic problems, and when the patient does not respond to treatment.

Therapy
Further diagnosis
Patient education

See specific diseases under Assessment.

TABLE 11-1
COMMON LOCATIONS OF SPECIFIC DERMATOSES

Nearly every dermatosis has particular areas of affinity. This can be an important diagnostic feature by indicating some conditions to be more likely than others.

LOCATION	DERMATOSES COMMONLY OCCURRING IN THIS AREA
Scalp	Seborrheic dermatitis, alopecia, psoriasis, furunculosis, eczema, sebaceous cysts, ringworm, pediculosis.
Ears	Seborrheic dermatitis, psoriasis, eczema, frostbite, basal cell or squamous cell carcinoma, contact dermatitis usually from hair dye.
Face	Acne, furunculosis, nevus, herpes simplex, ringworm, seborrheic dermatitis, milium, impetigo, erysipelas, lupus erythematosus, basal cell and squamous cell carcinoma, eczema, vitiligo.
Eyebrows	Seborrheic dermatitis, alopecia.
Eyelids	Eczema, contact dermatitis, milium, meibomian cyst, hordeolum.
Nose	Keratosis, carcinoma, furuncle, frostbite, tertiary syphilis.
Lips	Herpes simplex, contact dermatitis, leukoplakia, carcinoma, chancre.
Neck	Sebaceous cyst, furuncle, carbuncle, seborrheic dermatitis, contact dermatitis, ringworm, neurodermatitis, tinea versicolor.

271

Chest
: Acne, seborrheic dermatitis, tinea versicolor keratosis, herpes zoster, pityriasis rosea, eczema, psoriasis, scleroderma.

Axillae
: Furuncle, hyperhydrosis, contact dermatitis, seborrheic dermatitis, intertrigo, scabies, ringworm, molluscum contagiosum.

Forearms and wrists
: Keratosis pilaris, contact dermatitis, scabies, warts, erythema multiforme, lichen planus, occupational dermatitis.

Hands
: Warts, scabies, hyperhydrosis, contact dermatitis, eczema, syphilis (palms).

Back
: Acne, tinea versicolor, keratosis, herpes zoster, pediculosis, eczema, psoriasis, pityriasis rosea.

Abdomen
: Scabies, pediculosis corporis, urticaria, contact dermatitis, pityriasis rosea, tinea versicolor, eczema, herpes zoster, viral exanthemata, syphilis.

Buttocks
: Acne, furuncle, scabies, eczema, urticaria.

Gluteal crease and anus
: Eczema, condyloma latum, condyloma acuminatum (venereal wart), granuloma inguinale, lymphogranuloma venereum, seborrheic dermatitis, psoriasis.

Genitalia
: Chancre, chancroid, condyloma acuminatum, leukoplakia, moniliasis, scabies, pediculosis pubis, herpes simplex, lymphogranuloma, venereum, psoriasis.

Groin
: Tinea cruris, intertrigo, pediculosis corporis, granuloma inguinale, pityriasis rosea, seborrheic dermatitis, psoriasis.

Thighs	Scabies, keratosis pilaris, eczema, psoriasis, urticaria, exanthemata.
Knees and elbows	Psoriasis, xanthoma, scabies, atopic dermatitis.
Legs	Varicose ulcers, purpura, psoriasis, lichen planus, erythema nodosum, insect bites.
Feet	Tinea pedis, plantar wart, hyperhidrosis, callus, corn, contact dermatitis, frostbite, eczema, psoriasis, syphilis.

GLOSSARY

DEFINITION OF SKIN LESIONS*
PRIMARY LESIONS

Term		Description
Macule or Patch	<1 cm. >1 cm.	Circumscribed change in skin color which is not palpable.
Papule or Plaque	<1 cm. >1 cm.	Solid, elevated, palpable but superficial lesion.
Nodule or Tumor	<1 cm. >1 cm.	Solid lesion which may be elevated. They are palpable, and may be movable apart from adjacent structures.
Vesicle or Bulla	<1 cm. >1 cm.	Fluid-filled, elevated lesion.
Wheal		Evanescent lesion due to edema in the skin. Usually white or pale pink.
Comedo (blackhead)		Follicular plug of sebum and keratinous material.

*From Harvey et al.: The Principles and Practice of Medicine, 18th ed., 1972. Courtesy of Appleton-Century-Crofts, publishing division of Prentice-Hall, Inc.

Burrow

Linear, thread-like lesion (1 mm. to several cm.), slightly palpable.

SECONDARY LESIONS

Excoriation

Linear lesions secondary to trauma with loss of tissue.

Pustule

Elevated lesion, filled with purulent exudate, often follicular.

Abscess

Lesion below the surface of the skin, filled with purulent exudate.

Crust

Adherent, dried body fluid, as serum, blood, sebum or purulent exudate.

Fissure

Break in skin of varying depth, usually into upper dermis.

Scale

Dried plates of keratinized epithelial cells.

Lichenification

Accentuation of the normal skin markings accompanied by thickening.

Scar

Fibrotic healing of the dermis without normal skin appendages.

Atrophy

Loss of normal skin markings with thinning of the epidermis and/or dermis.

Ulcer

Depression formed by loss of superficial layers of skin.

GROUP CONFIGURATION OF SKIN LESIONS

Annular
  Arciform
  Polycyclic

Lesions arranged in circles, arcs or a combination thereof. Characteristic of drug eruptions, erythema multiforme, urticaria, psoriasis.

Serpiginous	Wavy lines–typical lesions of late syphilis.
Iris	Bull's-eye or target lesions. Characteristic of erythema multiforme.
Irregular	No distinctive pattern. Seen in urticaria, insect bites.
Zosteriform	Broad bands especially along nerve distribution as in herpes zoster.
Linear	Self-explanatory. Seen in lymphangitis, poison ivy dermatitis.

BIBLIOGRAPHY

Behrmann, H. T., et al.: *Common Skin Diseases*, 2nd ed., New York: Grune & Stratton, 1971.

Fitzpatrick, T. B., et al. (eds.): *Dermatology in General Medicine*, New York: McGraw Hill, 1971.

Harvey, A. M., et al.: *The Principles and Practice of Medicine*, 18th ed., New York: Appleton-Century-Crofts, 1972.

Johnson, S. A. M. (ed.): *The Skin and Internal Disease*, New York: McGraw Hill, 1967.

MacBryde, C. M. (ed.): *Signs and Symptoms*, 5th ed., Philadelphia: Lippincott, 1970.

Rook, A., D. S. Wilkinson, and F. J. G. Ebling: *Textbook of Dermatology*, Philadelphia: F. A. Davis Company, 1968.

Wintrobe, M. W., et al. (eds.): *Harrison's Principles of Internal Medicine*, 7th ed., New York: McGraw Hill, 1974.

NOTES

Chapter 12

Upper respiratory infection

UPPER RESPIRATORY INFECTION (URI) WORKSHEET

> To be used in patients with:
> Cold/Flu
> Sore Throat
> Runny Nose/Congestion
> Earache
> Cough

What you can't afford to miss: pneumonia, frontal sinusitis, bacterial meningitis, strep pharyngitis.

Chief Complaint:_____

SUBJECTIVE DATA:

Onset: _____Sudden _____Gradual _____Date

Course: _____Progressive _____Subsiding _____Same

Severity at worst: _____

Precipitated by:_____

Relieved by: _____

DESCRIBE POSITIVE RESPONSES
(Include Onset, Severity, Duration)

Yes   *No*

____ ____ Nasal symptoms:

_____Discharge: _____

_____White/clear

_____Purulent

_____Bloody

_____Congestion:_____

_____Postnasal drip: _____

_____Pain: _____

_____History of sinusitis:_____

_____History of hayfever:_____

_____Use of nosedrops more than 2 weeks:_____

_____Watery/itchy eyes: _____

____ ____ Throat/neck symptoms:

_____Sore throat:_____

_____Dysphagia: _____

_____Hoarseness: _____

_____Swollen glands (location):_____

_____Stiff neck: _____

____ ____ Ear symptoms:

_____Ache:_____

_____Drainage:_____

_____Serous

_____Purulent

_____Bloody

_____Past ear problems: _____

_____

_____Decreased hearing: _____

_____Exposure to noise/altitude

_____Tinnitus: _____

_____Vertigo:_____

_____Fullness/plugging: _____

____ ____ Chest Symptoms:

_____Cough: _____

_____Productive (color): _____

_____Nonproductive: _____

_____Worse at night:_____

_____Chest pain (location): _____

_____Pleuritic pain: _____

_____Shortness of breath:_____

_____History of asthma, chronic obstructive lung

disease, heart disease: _____

_____

_____Wheezing: _____

_____Ankle edema: _____

_____Paroxysmal nocturnal dyspnea:_____

_____Orthopnea:_____

_____Dyspnea on exertion:_____

ASSOCIATED WITH:
Yes   No

____ ____ Fever/chills: _____

____ ____ Night sweats:_____

____ ____ Muscle aches: _____

____ ____ Fatigue: _____

____ ____ Headache (location): _____

____ ____ Nausea/vomiting: _____

____ ____ Diarrhea:_____

____ ____ Rash:_____

____ ____ Dark urine:_____

____ ____ Other: _____

PAST MEDICAL HISTORY:
Yes   No

____ ____ Exposure to person with similar symptoms: _____

____ ____ Exposure to person with strep throat: _____

____ ____ Presently on medication: _____

_____

____ ____ Allergies (describe reaction): _____

____ ____ Smoker:
Amount: _____

____ ____ History of heart disease/rheumatic fever: _____

____ ____ History of heart murmur: _____

____ ____ History of chronic disease: _____

OBJECTIVE DATA:
Vital signs: _____B/P _____P _____R _____T _____Wt

General appearance: _____

DESCRIBE POSITIVE RESPONSES
Yes　*No*

____ ____ Rash: _____

NOSE EXAM: _____Not Done
(Examine if patient describes purulent or bloody drainage, has sinus tenderness, history of allergic rhinitis)
Yes　*No*

____ ____ Discharge: _____

____ ____ Mucosa abnormal:

_____Swollen: _____

_____Reddened: _____

_____Excoriation: _____

_____Polyp: _____

____ ____ Deviated septum:_____

____ ____ Sinus tenderness (note left or right):

_____Maxillary: _____

_____Frontal:_____

____ ____ Periorbital edema: _____

____ ____ Abnormal transillumination (note left or right):

_____Maxillary: _____

_____Frontal:_____

THROAT EXAM: _____Not Done

Yes _No_

____ ____ Red: _____

____ ____ Exudate: _____

____ ____ Vesicles: _____

____ ____ Membrane:_____

____ ____ Abnormal tonsils (note left or right):

_____Enlarged:_____

_____Exudate: _____

_____Abscess: _____

NECK EXAM: _____Not Done

Yes _No_

____ ____ Enlarged/tender nodes:_____

283

___ ___ Tender with flexion: _____

___ ___ Positive Kernig: _____

___ ___ Positive Brudzinski: _____

EAR EXAM: _____Not Done
Yes   No

___ ___ Abnormal external canal (note left or right):

_____Cerumen occludes: _____

_____Drainage:_____

_____Reddened: _____

_____Other: _____

___ ___ Abnormal tympanic membranes (note left or right):

_____Bulge: _____

_____Retracted: _____

_____Perforated: _____

_____Reddened: _____

_____Scarred: _____

_____Discharge: _____

_____Not visualized: _____

_____Other: _____

(If hearing decreased or ear exam abnormal, examine:)

___ ___ Abnormal Rinne: _____

___ ___ Abnormal Weber: Lateralization: ___Right ___Left

—— —— Gross hearing abnormal:

————Watch tick: _____

————Whispered word: _____

CHEST EXAM: _____Not Done
Yes   *No*

—— —— Rales: _____

—— —— Rhonchi: _____

—— —— Wheezes: _____

—— —— Dullness: _____

—— —— Altered fremitus: _____

—— —— Other: _____

ABDOMINAL EXAM: _____Not Done
Yes   *No*

—— —— Enlarged/tender liver: _____

—— —— Enlarged/tender spleen: _____

—— —— Masses: _____

—— —— Other: _____

CARDIAC EXAM: _____Not Done
Yes   *No*

—— —— Abnormal S_1/S_2: _____

—— —— Murmur: _____

—— —— Extra sounds: _____

—— —— Other: _____

LAB DATA (describe results):

Done Not
        Done

____ ____ CBC with differential: _____

____ ____ Chest x-ray:_____

____ ____ Sinus x-rays: _____

____ ____ Sputum gram stain: _____

____ ____ Arterial blood gases: _____

____ ____ Other: _____

ASSESSMENT:

_____

_____

_____

_____

PLAN:

_____ Admit: _____

DIAGNOSTIC:

                    Culture
          _____Beta strep screen

          _____Viral throat culture/serology

          _____Sputum culture

          _____Sputum for acid-fast bacilli

          _____Ear culture

          _____Nasal culture

_____Eye culture

Blood Work
_____CBC with differential

_____ESR

_____Mono spot test

_____Cold agglutinins

_____Liver function tests

_____Arterial blood gases

X-Ray
_____Chest: PA + Lateral

_____Sinus

_____Other_____

Other
_____Urinalysis

_____TB skin test:

_____Tine

_____PPD

THERAPEUTIC:

_____Antipyretic:_____

_____Analgesic: _____

_____Antibiotic: _____

_____Decongestant: _____

_____Antihistamine: _____

_____Cough suppressant/expectorant:_____

_____Lozenges/gargle: _____

_____Other: _____

PATIENT EDUCATION:

_____Force fluids: _____

_____Rest: _____

_____Humidifier:_____

_____Diet: _____

_____Stop smoking: _____

_____Return to clinic if symptoms persist: _____

_____Call for culture results: _____

_____Referral to other clinic: _____

_____Other: _____

UPPER RESPIRATORY INFECTION WORKSHEET RATIONALE

SUBJECTIVE DATA:

Onset	Helps differentiate acute from chronic process.
Course	New symptoms or change in symptoms can help in determining if the patient is developing a secondary bacterial infection, or is being infected by successive viral agents.
Severity at worst	Will help quantify the severity of the problem.

Precipitated by	May aid in determining the causative factors (e.g. allergic precipitants).
Relieved by	May also aid in identifying the etiology of the problem and in determining treatment.

Nasal Symptoms

Discharge Congestion	Inflammation of the mucous membranes leads to swelling, hyperemia, hypersecretion, and may cause nasal obstruction.
White/clear	May indicate viral or allergic etiology.
Purulent	Caused by presence of leukocytes, and indicates viral or bacterial etiology.
Bloody	May be due to a local cause such as coughing, sneezing, injury, or may be secondary to nose picking, ulcerations; may accompany polyps or acute infections.
Postnasal drip	Occurs with anterior nasal obstruction. May irritate throat, resulting in soreness or stimulation of cough reflex.
Face/head/jaw/tooth pain	Indicates sinusitis due to impairment of drainage by the boggy, engorged nasal mucosa resulting in increased tension within the sinus. Pain is referred to areas of the 5th cranial nerve. With sinusitis involving:

Frontal: pain is over frontal sinuses.

Maxillary: pain is over maxillary sinuses and teeth.

Ethmoid and sphenoid: pain is between and behind eyes.

History of sinusitis	Helps to determine if chronic sinusitis is present.
History of hay fever (allergic rhinitis)	Presenting symptoms may represent an allergic flare-up.
	Patients with hay fever are more susceptible to irritants and infection. If persistent, may develop into sinusitis or nasal polyps.
Use of nose drops for more than 2 weeks	Prolonged use of local vasoconstrictive medication disposes to a chronic congestive state, due to a rebound phenomenon.
Watery/itchy eyes	May represent systemic infection (e.g. viremia), local infection (e.g. conjunctivitis) or allergy.

Throat/Neck Symptoms

Sore throat	Indicates inflammation of highly sensitive pharyngeal mucous membranes or irritation from postnasal drip, cough, mouth breathing.
Dysphagia	Is related to the degree of pharyngeal swelling, presence of ulceration or lymphadenopathy.
Hoarseness	Is a sign of infection or inflammation of larynx, primarily viral.
Swollen glands	Indicates a response to infection. Regional adenopathy occurs with a

localized infection and generalized adenopathy with a systemic infection.

Stiff neck

May indicate meningitis with acute subarachnoid suppuration. Patient keeps neck extended to reduce the stretch on inflamed spinal structures.

Ear Symptoms
Ache

May indicate inflammation/ infection of the external or middle ear; may be due to only partial closure of the eustachian tube with inflammation from the pharynx.

Drainage

Suggests infection:

External otitis: bloody, watery, purulent.
Acute or chronic otitis media with perforation: purulent.
Mastoiditis: purulent.
Cholesteatoma: very foul-smelling; dirty grayish yellow.

Past ear problems

Suggests chronic otitis media and alerts one to watch for complications.

Decreased hearing

Suggests impaction, external obstruction, swelling, conductive or sensorineural hearing loss.

Tinnitus

Accompanies hearing loss, disorders of the external, middle or inner ear or of the auditory nerve. Is presumed to be due to irritation of nerve endings in the cochlea by degenerative, vascular or vasomotor disease.

	May also be due to aspirin toxicity.
Vertigo	Is caused by inflammation of the labyrinth.
Fullness	Results from negative pressure in the middle ear due to closure of the eustachian tubes.

Chest Symptoms

Cough	Is produced by inflammatory or mechanical stimulation upon nerve endings of the vagus nerve in the pharynx, larynx or trachea. It is a protective reflex intended to clear the airway.
Productive:	
White/clear	Associated with viral infection.
Purulent	Associated with viral or bacterial infection.
Blood streaked	May be secondary to inflammation in the nose, pharynx, gums, larynx, or to paroxysms of coughing and trauma to mucosa.
Blood	Associated with tuberculosis, lung abscess, bronchiectasis, pulmonary infarction, cancer and any erosion of the bronchioles.
Worse at night	Secretions are not being removed as frequently as during the day, and accumulate and provoke cough. May be secondary to a postnasal drip which increases in a reclining position.
Chest pain	Thoracic movement displaces irritated rib, muscle, nerves and pleural surfaces causing pain.

Pleuritic pain	Pain is secondary to stretching of the inflamed parietal pleura.
Shortness of breath	Indicates a severe pharyngeal swelling and/or obstruction in the airways.
History of asthma/chronic obstructive lung disease/ heart disease	
Wheezing	Occurs with airway narrowing secondary to bronchospasm or secretions.
Ankle edema Paroxysmal nocturnal dyspnea Orthopnea Dyspnea on exertion	Fever, tachycardia and hypoxemia increase metabolic demands and place a further burden on the overloaded but compensated myocardium of patients with heart disease; this may precipitate heart failure.

Associated with

Fever/chills	Indicates systemic infection. Rigor (shaking chills) is typical of a pyogenic infection with bacteremia.
Night sweats	Associated with tuberculosis or intermittent fever spikes.
Muscle aches	It is not known if this reflects the presence of an infectious agent, or if it is merely a nonspecific accompaniment of pyrexia.
Fatigue	A nonspecific symptom associated with a variety of viral infections or chronic bacterial infections.
Headache	May indicate sinusitis/meningitis, or may be a nonspecific accompaniment of a viral infection.

Nausea/vomiting/diarrhea	Associated with gastroenteritis.
Rash	May indicate a viral or bacterial illness. See Assessment.
Dark urine	May be a sign of hepatitis caused by infectious mononucleosis with bilirubinuria (impaired excretion of bilirubin by the liver).

Past Medical History

Exposure to person with similar symptoms	Helps to explain etiology by identifying predisposing contacts.
Exposure to person with strep throat	
Present medications	This information is necessary to determine what the patient has tried and if it's working.
Allergies	Will influence choice of treatment. May also be the source of the patient's problem.
Smoking	Cigarette smoke inhibits ciliary movement and macrophage activity in the lungs, and may thus prolong the duration of the infection.
History of heart disease/ rheumatic fever	It is important to prevent recurrent rheumatic fever, especially with valve damage, by early vigorous treatment of a strep infection.
	Patients with a history of rheumatic fever are more apt to have a recurrence with a strep infection than is the general population.
History of heart murmur	It is important to determine this in patients without a known history of rheumatic fever who may have had

it, with a resultant heart murmur (usually that of mitral stenosis).

History of chronic disease — It may be a predisposing factor which increases susceptibility to infection.

OBJECTIVE DATA:
Vital signs
    Blood pressure
    Respirations/Pulse
    Temperature

Are indicators of the patient's general status. Fever and tachycardia are usually present with a systemic infection.

General appearance

Usually helpful in assessing the degree of illness.

Rash

Viral causes and appearances of rash:

Infectious mononucleosis: maculopapular, resembles rubella, is rarely papulovesicular.
Enterovirus: maculopapular, resembles rubella, rarely papulovesicular or petechial.
Rubeola: maculopapular, bright red, begins on the head and neck and spreads downward.
Rubella: maculopapular, pink, begins on the head and neck and spreads downward.

Bacterial causes and appearances of rash:

Meningococcemia: maculopapular and petechial.
Scarlet fever: generalized, punctate, red, prominent on neck.

295

Nose Exam

Discharge	Observe quality. See Subjective Data.
Mucosal changes	Mucosa is reddened and swollen with inflammation or infection.
Polyp	Is hypertrophy of mucosa from recurrent episodes of mucosal edema; frequently from longstanding rhinitis; may enlarge to obstruct air passage.
Deviated septum	Cartilaginous and bony septum may encroach upon the nasal chamber and sinus ostia and cause obstruction.
Sinus tenderness Maxillary Frontal	May indicate sinusitis.
Periorbital edema	Infection may extend from the paranasal sinus spaces through the venous network. This is the first sign of extension of infection into the orbit.
Transillumination	This is a technique of undocumented usefulness. Decreased light transmission may indicate mucosal thickening or the presence of fluid.

Throat Exam

Reddened	Is a sign of inflammation.
Exudate	Associated with strep, adenovirus, mononucleosis, Vincent's angina, diphtheria and herpes simplex.
Vesicles	Associated with viral infections; e.g. herpes simplex.

296

Membrane	Presence is associated with diphtheria.
Enlarged tonsils	Is a sign of inflammation with accumulation of leukocytes, dead epithelial cells and pathogenic bacteria in the crypts.
Peritonsillar abscess	Infection spreads to the peritonsillar space, deep to the tonsil, and the swelling pushes the tonsil and tonsillar pillar toward or across the midline. Swelling often extends to the soft palate and the uvula is displaced.

Neck Exam
Enlarged/tender nodes	Enlarged anterior cervical triangle nodes are more common with bacterial infections and mononucleosis. Posterior cervical nodes are more commonly enlarged in viral infections (rubella). Posterior auricular and occipital nodes are more commonly involved with rubella and infectious mononucleosis.
Tender with flexion/ nuchal rigidity Positive Kernig Positive Brudzinski	Associated with meningitis. Results from inflamed meninges with reflex muscular spasm.

Ear Exam
External canal
Drainage	May be secondary to infection (fungal or bacterial), dermatitis or furuncle.
Tympanic membrane: Reddened/bulge/ retracted/perforated	May bulge with acute otitis media due to pressure of retained secretions. Is retracted with serous otitis

media; amber color and air bubbles or fluid may be seen. In otitis media, the tympanic membrane is first reddened due to dilation of blood vessels, followed by diffuse dullness, hyperemia and loss of landmarks.

Scarring

Reflects previous ear infections or perforation.

Discharge

May occur secondary to acute perforation, chronic otitis with cholesteatoma.

Rinne

Tests hearing perception and conduction. Air conduction normally is twice as long as bone conduction.

Weber

Lateralization of the sound to one ear indicates a conductive loss in that ear or a perceptive loss in the opposite ear. A conductive hearing loss (never marked) occurs with acute otitis media or serous otitis media.

Chest Exam
Rales

Originate in the alveoli, and are associated with pneumonia and congestive heart failure.

Rhonchi

These are equivalent to coarse rales, and originate in the large airways (trachea, bronchi).

Wheezes

Are due to airway narrowing, bronchospasm. Associated with asthma, foreign bodies and mucus.

Dullness

Associated with atelectasis, pneumonia and pleural effusion.

Altered fremitus	Egophony; E-A changes are found in consolidation and effusion. Tactile fremitus is increased with consolidation in pneumonia or with inflammation around a lung abscess. It is decreased with pleural thickening, pleural effusion or pneumothorax.
Abdominal Exam	Indicated if infectious mononucleosis is suspected. Enlarged spleen is often present.

Cardiac Exam

Murmur	May be associated with valvular disease due to rheumatic fever.
Extra sounds	Associated with heart disease.

Lab Data

CBC with differential	Helps to determine infection. Will show: leukocytosis with bacterial infections; leukopenia and lymphocytosis (large atypical lymphs) with viral infection; monocytosis with typhoid, tuberculosis, subacute bacterial endocarditis; eosinophilia may imply underlying allergic disorder.
Chest x-ray	To determine presence of infiltrates, effusion, lobar consolidation, abscesses, mass lesions, pulmonary infarcts, etc.
Sinus x-ray	Helps to determine sinusitis with mucosal thickening, opacification, or air fluid levels.
Sputum gram stain	Helps identify specific pathogens in pneumonia.

Arterial blood gases

Hypoxia may be present in pneumonia.

ASSESSMENT:

The term "upper respiratory infection" encompasses several symptom complexes including infections of the ear, nose and throat. The most common cause is a virus. Viral respiratory diseases are responsible for ½ or more of all acute illnesses. The influenza virus is the only agent among them which causes significant mortality in adults. URI's are associated with a spectrum of host responses, varying from asymptomatic carriers to severe and sometimes fatal pneumonias. A few clinical and epidemiologic entities can be recognized without laboratory tests, but the causative agent in a large proportion of cases cannot be identified without virologic studies.

150 serotypes, representing 12 groups of viruses, have been associated with respiratory disease in humans.

Viruses cause ¾ or more of acute respiratory illnesses; ½ of these are due to rhinovirus. The principal nonviral causes are *M. pneumoniae* and hemolytic streptococcus.

Common cold

The common cold consists of nasal congestion, discharge, sneezing, moderate sore throat, mild constitutional symptoms, usually without fever. In adults, ⅔ of these are caused by rhinovirus, respiratory syncytial virus and coronaviruses.

Rhinovirus

Incubation period 1-5 days; symptoms last about 3 days. Rarely causes bronchitis in adults, but occurs commonly in children.

Respiratory syncytial virus

Incubation period is 5 days; symptoms last about 3 days. Occasionally progresses to bacterial sinusitis.

Coronavirus

Incubation period 3-5 days; short duration of symptoms.

Adenovirus

Produces several major patterns of illness:

1. Acute respiratory disease (ARD). Affects military recruits; seen in only 2 % of civilians. It is a febrile illness, lasting about 1 week with pharyngitis, cough, hoarseness, and may extend to atypical pneumonia.

2. Febrile pharyngitis. Little or no exudate. Lasts 5-6 days.

3. Pharyngoconjunctival fever with nonpurulent conjunctivitis. Lasts 5-6 days.

Parainfluenza

Incubation period 5-6 days.

It is more severe and serious in infants and children, causing laryngotracheal bronchitis and croup. In adults, it produces "cold," hoarseness and cough. Complications include bacterial sinusitis; in patients with chronic lung disease, pulmonary bacterial superinfection should be considered.

Coxsackie virus

Occurs more commonly in the summer. There may be multiple recurrent infections within a family, with varying manifestations.

Coxsackie A

Herpangina (small papular, vesicular or ulcerative lesions on anterior pillars, tonsils, pharynx); lymphoid pharyngitis (raised, discrete, white/yellow papules surrounded by erythema on uvula, pillars, pharynx); upper and lower respiratory disease; cutaneous eruptions, hepatitis, aseptic meningitis.

Coxsackie B

Upper respiratory infection, exanthems, diarrhea, pleurodynia, orchitis, pneumonia, hemolytic-uremic syndrome, cardiac and central nervous system disease.

Nasal discharge/congestion

In the course of warming, humidifying and cleansing inspired air, the nasopharynx is exposed to a multitude of irritants and infectious agents. The lining membrane contains many mucous glands and deposits of lymphoid tissue. Engorgement, hypersecretion of mucus, hyperplasia of the adenoids and other lymphatic foci occur in response to irritation or infection, and can produce acute or chronic obstruction of the passages draining the sinuses, conjunctiva and middle ear. This leads to initiation or aggravation of bacterial infection in these areas.

Sinusitis

This is an acute, usually bacterial infection initiated by impairment of drainage by the boggy, engorged nasal mucosa of allergic or viral rhinitis. It may also be secondary to dental infection in 10 % of cases.

Occasionally, air travel with pressure changes, or deviations of the nasal septum, are contributory. Symptoms include: local pain and tenderness, sometimes with edema of the overlying facial skin; headache; occasionally fever. The headache is worse in the morning when exudate has accumulated overnight, and tends to improve with upright posture and drainage during the day. It is commonly caused by *D. pneumoniae, H. influenzae, group A streptococcus and S. aureus*. Complications are rare, but may be serious. Frank suppuration and abscess may lead to osteomyelitis and spread of infection to the orbit, meninges or brain. Repeated episodes of acute infections lead to thickening of the sinus mucosa, continued partial obstruction and chronic inflammation that easily flares up. Each acute episode becomes more difficult to control. Intensive treatment of acute exacerbations will bring relief, but surgery may eventually be necessary to ensure free drainage. Distinctions among acute, chronic and inactive disease may be impossible radiologically. The diagnosis must then depend on the patient's symptoms as well as on bacterial cultures of sinus aspirates.

Allergic rhinitis

This consists of sneezing, rhinorrhea, swelling of the nasal mucosa, itchy eyes and lacrimation. Hay fever is due to the seasonal spread of pollen in the air, but similar symptoms may be caused by exposure to antigens other than pol-

303

len. Infections of the sinuses and middle ear are common complications of perennial allergic rhinitis, but are uncommon in seasonal hay fever. Infections of the sinuses or nose in patients with allergic rhinitis lead to nasal polyps which further obstruct nasal passages, increase symptoms and exaggerate infection. Studies indicate that the nasal mucosa of patients with allergic rhinitis is more susceptible to viral respiratory infections.

Sore throat

May be caused by bacteria or virus. The major bacterial cause is the streptococcus, and the incubation period is 3-5 days. It begins abruptly and is associated with headache, fever (102°-104° F.) and chills. Symptoms reach maximum intensity within 24-48 hours. Nasal congestion and discharge and cough are minor complaints, and loss of voice does not occur. There may be otalgia present in the form of referred pain. With fever, there may be a blush to the skin, and when this is pronounced, a diagnosis of scarlet fever is made. Various degrees of redness and edema of the mucous membranes of the posterior pharynx and tonsils are present. Characteristically, there is discrete to confluent exudate on the tonsils with anterior cervical adenopathy and leukocytosis. A throat culture should be done; there may be 3-10 % negative growth even in the presence of strep. The beta hemolytic group A strain is the only one that has conclusively been associated with rheumatic fever and glomerulonephritis. The incidence of glomerulonephritis has not been shown to be influenced by treatment. The 3 % incidence of acute rheumatic fever after strep infection in general applies to epidemics of virulent M—typeable group A strep in highly susceptible individuals. Sporadic strep infections in the general population have been reported to cause acute rheumatic fever (ARF) at rates of 0-1 %. ARF can be prevented even if treatment is delayed up to ten days.

Peritonsillar abscess

May occur early or late in the course of an acute tonsillitis, and is usually unilateral. It is associated with marked dysphagia, pain, increased salivation, trismus. The patient speaks with difficulty and has a temperature around 100° F. Abscess formation requires surgical drainage and intravenous antibiotic therapy.

Vincent's angina

This condition has an insidious onset without constitutional symptoms, so that fever is rare. Exudate is present with little surrounding inflammation, and generally involves one tonsil with unilateral cervical adenopathy.

Diphtheria

Has a gradual onset without severe symptoms. Sore throat is not a constant feature. The exudate is smooth, cream-colored and appears to be incorporated in the mucous membrane. It is hard to remove, leaving a bleeding bed.

Adenovirus

Causes URI symptoms and exudative lesions with constitutional symptoms. The onset is less rapid, with mild sore throat, hoarseness and cough. The exudate is rarely confluent, and the lymph nodes are only slightly tender.

Infectious mononucleosis

Has an insidious onset and malaise is prominent. Exudate is present 50 % of the time, and the fever is more prolonged than with strep throat. Lymph node enlargement is generalized, and the spleen may be palpable. A fleeting skin rash may be seen or reported 10-15 % of the time.

Herpes simplex I

Has an incubation period of 2-12 days. Produces gingivostomatitis, fever, irritability, vesicular eruption on the mucous membrane, submaxillary or anterior cervical adenopathy. Vesicles rupture and produce small ulcers covered with exudate. They are scattered throughout the mucous membranes of the mouth, and a "kissing ulcer" under the tip of the tongue is typical.

Rash
  Rubeola

Initial symptoms include malaise, irritability, fever as high as 105° F., conjunctivitis, excessive lacrimation, eyelid edema, photophobia, hacking cough, nasal discharge, Koplik spots (small red, irregular lesions with blue-white centers, which appear on the mucous membranes 1-2 days before the rash). The rash is bright red, maculopapular, spreads from forehead to face, neck and trunk and lasts about 6 days.

Rubella

The prodrome preceding the exanthem lasts 1-7 days with malaise, headache, fever, mild conjunctivitis and lymphadenopathy. The rash is maculopapular, pink, begins on the forehead and face and spreads downward to the trunk and extremities. It is commonly present for 3 days. In pregnancy the disease may lead to serious fetal disorders.

Earache
  External otitis

Produces itching and pain with a dry, scaly ear canal. There may be a watery, bloody or purulent discharge with intermediate deafness. There are 3 main types:

1. *Furuncle:* begins in the pilosebaceous follicle, secondary to a strep infection.

2. *Fungal or bacterial:* mainly involving staphylococcus and gram-negative rods.

3. *Dermatitis:* consisting of eczema, contact dermatitis or seborrhea. Frequently secondary to warm, moist climates, swimming, bathing or trauma through cleaning or scratching.

  Serous otitis media

Partial or complete closure of the eustachian tube results in negative pressure in the middle ear, causing transudation of serum into the middle ear. This produces symptoms of hearing loss or a full, plugged feeling. This is caused by:

1. Inflammation of the pharynx or infected lymphoid tissue.

2. An allergic reaction.

3. Sudden changes in atmospheric pressure.

Acute otitis media

Follows or accompanies a URI. The acute inflammation of the middle ear mucosa leads to suppuration and often perforation. Usually it is secondary to staphylococcal or pneumococcal infection. The patient complains of fullness and pressure in the ears and fever and chills.

Chronic otitis media

Is nearly always associated with perforation of the eardrum. It is usually the result of one of the following developments:

1. A severe infection, causing necrotic changes in some portion of the tympanic membrane. Today this seems to be a relatively rare occurrence.

2. An acute inflammation in which the tympanic membrane is hyperplastic or fibrotic, with a limited capacity to heal.

3. The formation of a cholesteatoma subsequent to an ingrowth of squamous epithelium through a marginal tympanic perforation.

Complications include:

1. *Mastoiditis:* The inflammation has extended through the cortex of the mastoid process. Occurrence

indicated by postaural edema, tenderness, ear drainage and sepsis.

2. *Labyrinthitis:* Erosion of the bony, horizontal semicircular canal by a cholesteatoma exposes the membranous labyrinth.

3. *Meningitis:* Extension of the infection through the lateral sinus from an extradural abscess.

4. *Brain abscess:* Apt to follow a lateral sinus thrombophlebitis, petrositis (inflammation of the petrous portion of the temporal bone) or meningitis.

Acute nonsuppurative labyrinthitis	Usually secondary to a URI. Consists of vertigo, marked tinnitus, staggering gait and nystagmus without hearing loss.
Decreased hearing	Due to either a conductive or a sensorineural loss. Conductive loss may be due to:

1. Obstruction to the passage of sound waves through the external auditory canal, as with impacted cerumen and external otitis (occlusion with edema and debris).

2. Abnormalities of the tympanic membrane, such as excessive thickening, retraction or perforation. With marked changes in the tympanic membrane, an abnormal middle ear condition exists which is also a factor.

3. Pathologic changes in the middle ear which interfere with mobil-

ity of the ossicular chain, including fixation of ossicular joints, tympanosclerotic changes, secretions and granulation tissue.

4. Pathologic changes in the capsule of the labyrinth causing a fixation of the oval window (otosclerosis).

Sensorineural loss includes:

1. *Presbycusis:* High tone loss which develops in everyone in time, due to aging atrophy.

2. *Acoustic trauma:* Noise exposure (with degeneration of the organ of Corti), exposure to blasts (which ruptures the drumhead or displaces the organ of Corti), blows to the head (which occlude the meatus, resulting in transmitted pressure to the perforated drumhead).

Meningitis

Usually occurs after a viral URI, pneumococcal infection of the sinus or lung, or, by extension, infection from surface structures.

Symptoms include fever, headache, vomiting, confusion, delirium, convulsions, petechial rash of the skin and mucous membranes, neck and back stiffness with positive Kernig's and Brudzinski's signs on physical exam. The cause may be bacterial or viral.

Bacterial

Bacterial or purulent meningitis in adults is due to infection with meningococci (40 %), pneumococci, streptococci or staphylococci.

Meningococcal: Results from a bacteremia originating in a nasopharyngeal focus, and localizing in the meninges. Spread by respiratory droplets from persons with mild upper respiratory infections and mainly by healthy carriers. 38 % carrier incidence has been observed during epidemics.

Pneumococcal: Preceding infection usually is present, and a focus is often demonstrated in the lungs.

Streptococcal, Staphylococcal: Occur in the middle ear or sinuses and spread to the meninges.

Viral

Due to viruses of the following types: arthropod-borne encephalitis, lymphocytic choriomeningitis, mumps, rabies, infectious mononucleosis, herpes simplex, Coxsackie or ECHO virus infections.

Acute bronchitis

Characterized by a productive (mucopurulent or purulent) cough and the absence of x-ray densities. On exam, musical rhonchi are commonly heard and wheezing is occasionally present. It is common in viral infections in healthy adults and is rarely serious.

Sputum cultures are usually sterile (transtracheal aspirate) but may reveal pneumococci or beta hemolytic strep. Antibiotics are used in an attempt to prevent secondary infection in patients with impaired respiratory or cardiac function or debilitating illness. Some studies show them to shorten the course.

Pneumonia

An inflammation in the lung parenchyma, most commonly caused by infection. Pneumococcus accounts for 80 % or more of the primary bacterial infections. A URI may predispose one to pneumonia.

Onset is usually sudden with shaking chills, "stabbing" chest pain, fever and productive cough.

Klebsiella
Pseudomonas } Pneumonia
Proteus

Occur mainly in persons between 40-60 years old with a history of alcoholism, malnutrition or debilitating disease. They are also a frequent type of superinfection in persons hospitalized for serious disease, including other types of pneumonia treated with antibiotics.

Hemophilus influenza: Rare in adults. Has occurred in the presence of cardiac disease, chronic obstructive pulmonary disease and hypogammaglobulinemia.

Streptococcus: Usually occurs as a sequel to viral URI's, especially influenza or measles, or in persons with underlying pulmonary disease. Patients are severely toxic and cyanotic. Pleural effusion develops frequently and early and progresses to empyema in ⅓ of untreated cases.

Staphylococcus: Usually occurs as a sequal to viral URI's, especially influenza, and in debilitated patients.

PPLO (pleuropneumonia-like organism)
Mycoplasma pneumonia/ viral pneumonia

Has an intrafamilial spread; is rare in those over 40. It has an incubation period of 9-12 days and causes a URI. A small percentage develop bronchitis and pneumonia. A cough, which may be blood-flecked, is universal, but gross hemoptysis is rare. Harsh or diminished breath sounds and fine inspiratory rales involving bilateral lower lobes are frequently found. If untreated, complications are rare.

Mycoplasma may also involve the ear, causing congestion of the tympanic membrane and a bullous myringitis.

PLAN:
Admit

Bacterial meningitis; frontal sinusitis; most pneumonias.

Diagnostic
Culture
B strep screen

To document the presence of beta hemolytic strep, group A.

Viral culture/serology

To isolate viruses to determine etiology of symptoms.

Sputum culture

To identify causative organism.

Sputum for acid-fast bacilli

To identify tuberculosis bacilli.

Ear culture
Nasal culture
Eye culture

To identify specific pathogens.

313

Blood work

CBC with differential	See Lab Data. White blood count and differential help in separating viral and bacterial infections.
ESR (erythrocyte sedimentation rate)	Is a nonspecific indicator of disease; is increased in infection, degenerative, neoplastic and collagen diseases.
Mono spot test	To aid in diagnosing infectious mononucleosis.
Cold agglutinins	Is positive for mycoplasma.
Liver function tests	To determine the presence of hepatitis. May be elevated in mononucleosis.
Arterial blood gases	To determine changes in oxygen concentration.
Chest x-ray Sinus x-ray	To aid in determining the extent and site of infection.
Urinalysis	To determine the presence of bilirubin.
TB skin test	To rule out tuberculosis.
Referral to other clinics	Usually for persistent infection or diagnostic problems. Otolaryngologist may be helpful in many instances.

Therapeutic

Antipyretic	Aspirin or acetaminophen (Tylenol) will reduce fever; also provides symptomatic relief for myalgias.
Analgesic	Provides symptomatic relief.
Antibiotic	To treat infections. The initial choice of drug may be based on the

most likely causative organism and subsequently changed on the basis of culture and sensitivity reports.

Decongestant

Has an indirect sympathomimetic effect as mucous membrane decongestant by releasing norepinephrine.

Antihistamine

May decrease inflammatory response; dries secretions and usually induces sleep or sedation.

Cough expectorant

Effectiveness has not been established.

Cough suppressant

Helpful if cough keeps patient awake at night. Should *not* be given if patient has copious secretions, as secretions may collect rather than be expectorated.

Lozenges/gargle

Help relieve pharyngeal irritation and decrease pharyngeal muscle spasm.

Patient education
Force fluids

To avoid dehydration, especially if temperature is elevated; also helps loosen secretions.

Rest

Important until systemic symptoms subside.

Humidifier

To relieve airway irritation due to drying.

Diet

Encourage liquids if patient has pharyngitis, soft foods with gastroenteritis.

Smoking

Emphasize irritating effects on mucosa and aggravation of symptoms. It may also prolong course of cough.

315

BIBLIOGRAPHY

Boies, Lawrence R., Jerome A. Helger, and Robert E. Priest: *Fundamentals of Otolaryngology*, 4th ed., Philadelphia: Saunders, 1964.

DeGowin, Elmer, and Richard DeGowin: *Bedside Diagnostic Examination*, 2nd ed., London: Macmillan, 1969.

Krupp, Marcus A., and Milton J. Chatton: *Current Diagnosis and Treatment*, Los Altos: Lange Medical Publications, 1972.

MacBryde, C. M. (ed.): *Signs and Symptoms*, 5th ed., Philadelphia: Lippincott, 1970.

Wintrobe, Maxwell M., et al.: *Harrison's Principles of Internal Medicine*, 7th ed., New York: McGraw Hill, 1974.

NOTES

NOTES

Chapter 13

Vaginal discharge

VAGINAL DISCHARGE WORKSHEET

To be used for patients with:
Vaginal Discharge
Genital Itching
Females with Venereal Disease
Females with Burning on Urination

What you can't afford to miss: gonorrhea, ectopic pregnancy.

Chief Complaint:_____
SUBJECTIVE DATA:

DESCRIBE POSITIVE RESPONSES
(Include Onset, Severity, Duration, Location)

Yes   *No*

___ ___ Vaginal discharge: _____

___ ___ Sores: _____

___ ___ Rash:_____

___ ___ Genital itching or burning: _____

___ ___ Abdominal pain: _____

Protocols for Common Acute Self-Limiting Problems

___ ___ Fever and chills: _____

___ ___ Achy joints with present illness: _____

___ ___ Nausea and vomiting:_____

___ ___ Dyspareunia: _____

___ ___ Contact with someone with venereal disease:

Type of venereal disease and evidence for it: _____

_____

___ ___ Birth control:

_____Birth control pills

How long: _____

_____Intrauterine device

How long: _____

_____Condom

_____Diaphragm

_____Other: _____

___ ___ Does patient douche?: _____

___ ___ Use of feminine hygiene sprays: _____

___ ___ Current and recent antibiotic therapy: _____

Date of last menstrual period:_____

PROBLEMS WITH URINATION:
Yes *No*

___ ___ Frequency:_____

—— —— Urgency: _____

—— —— Dysuria: _____

—— —— Hematuria: _____

—— —— Odor: _____

—— —— Cloudy urine: _____

—— —— Other: _____

PAST MEDICAL HISTORY:
Yes   *No*

—— —— Hospitalization or history of serious illness: _____

_____

—— —— Diabetes mellitus in patient or family members: _____

_____

—— —— History of venereal disease:

        Treatment: _____

—— —— Previous vaginal infections: _____

ALLERGIES: (specify reaction)
Yes   *No*

—— —— Penicillin: _____

—— —— Sulfa: _____

—— —— Tetracycline: _____

—— —— Other: _____

OBJECTIVE DATA:

Vital signs: _____B/P _____P _____R _____T

PELVIC EXAM: _____Not Done

Yes *No*

____ ____ Inflammation of Bartholin's and Skene's glands:_____

____ ____ Sores or rashes:_____

____ ____ Venereal warts: _____

____ ____ Urethra reddened: _____

____ ____ Urethra swollen: _____

____ ____ Vaginal lesions:_____

____ ____ Injection of vaginal mucosa: _____

____ ____ Discharge: _____

____ ____ Foul odor: _____

____ ____ Cervical erosion: _____

____ ____ Discharge from cervical os: _____

____ ____ Cervical tenderness: _____

____ ____ Mass or fullness: _____

____ ____ Adnexal masses or tenderness: _____

____ ____ Inguinal adenopathy: _____

ABDOMINAL EXAM: _____Not Done

_____

LAB DATA:
*Done Not
        Done*

—— —— CBC: _____

—— —— ESR: _____

—— —— Wet prep:_____

—— —— KOH prep: _____

—— —— Gravindex: _____Negative _____Positive

—— —— Urinalysis: _____

—— —— Other: _____

ASSESSMENT:

_____ Monilial vaginitis

_____ Trichomonal vaginitis

_____ Gonorrhea

_____ GC. contact

_____ Nonspecific vaginitis

_____ Herpes progenitalis

_____ Other:_____

THERAPY:
_____ No Rx

_____ Rx deferred pending test results

Protocols for Common Acute Self-Limiting Problems

_____ Antibiotics: _____

_____ Suppositories: _____

_____ Analgesics: _____

_____ Other: _____

PLAN:
Done Not
      Done

____ ____ Gonorrhea culture:

             Call for results: _____

             Date: _____

____ ____ VDRL: _____

____ ____ Blood glucose: _____

____ ____ Admit to hospital: _____

____ ____ Gynecology consult: _____

PATIENT EDUCATION:

_____ Return if no improvement: _____

_____ Call for results of culture: _____

_____ Return for reculture: _____

_____ Proper use of suppositories: _____

_____ Other: _____

VAGINAL DISCHARGE WORKSHEET RATIONALE

SUBJECTIVE DATA:

Vaginal Discharge	Indicates gonococcal, monilial, trichomonal or nonspecific vaginitis.
Character of discharge	Frequently gives strong clue to causative organism. However, is not always pathognomonic.
Curd-like	Characteristic of moniliasis.
Greenish-yellow, frothy	Characteristic of trichomoniasis; discharge is vaginal, not cervical, in origin.
Gray and homogeneous	Characteristic of nonspecific or hemophilus vaginitis.
Greenish or purulent	Characteristic of gonococcal discharge; is cervical in origin.
Sores	May be indicative of primary syphilis (chancre) or herpes progenitalis. Sores and excoriation may be secondary to scratching with resulting abrasions.
Rash	May be indicative of secondary syphilis or rash associated with gonococcemia.
Genital Itching or Burning	May occur secondary to irritation of labia, vagina and urethra by vaginal discharge.
Abdominal Pain	Usually occurs with salpingitis secondary to gonococcal infection, or secondary to ectopic pregnancy.

Fever and Chills	Usually occurs with salpingitis or disseminated gonococcal infection; implies bacterial infection.
Aching Joints with Present Illness	May indicate gonococcemia. Initially, consists of arthralgias and may proceed to tenosynovitis and arthritis involving several joints asymmetrically.
Nausea and Vomiting	May be indicative of extension of gonococcal infection into pelvis with resulting abscess.
Dyspareunia	May occur with herpes progenitalis, moniliasis, trichomoniasis or gonorrhea. It is secondary to irritation of the perineum and vaginal mucosa or peritoneal irritation in disseminated gonorrhea.
Contact with Person with Venereal Disease	Syphilis and gonorrhea are transmitted by sexual intercourse. Trichomoniasis is also believed to be transmitted sexually and some sources classify it as a venereal disease.
Method of birth control Birth control pills	Birth control pills increase the glycogen content of vaginal epithelium which serves as a good medium for monilia.
Intrauterine device	The intrauterine device (IUD) is considered a foreign body in the uterus. It causes local irritation, and some women may develop endometritis. An IUD should not be inserted in women with a history of salpingitis.

Condom

This is the only method of contraception that may help prevent venereal disease.

Diaphragm

Local reactions may occur due to the gel or foam used concurrently.

Frequency of douching

Douching can decrease the acidity of the vagina; the pH change may induce vaginitis, especially trichomonal.

Feminine hygiene sprays

These have been associated with contact dermatitis and milder local irritation.

Antibiotic Therapy

Changes the normal vaginal flora and allows bacterial or fungal overgrowth, with resulting vaginitis.

Date of last menstrual period

Trichomoniasis and gonorrhea frequently occur or are exacerbated after menses. Date of menses is also important to rule out possibility of pregnancy. Incidence of trichomoniasis is increased in pregnancy.

Problems with urination
Frequency

May be caused by inflammation of urethra secondary to herpes simplex II, trichomoniasis, moniliasis or gonorrhea. It may be indicative of diabetes mellitus (polyuria) or urinary tract infection.

Dysuria

Caused by inflammation of the urethra secondary to gonorrhea or vulvar irritation. See Dysuria Protocol.

Urgency, hematuria, cloudy urine

See Dysuria Protocol.

Foul odor

Indicates overgrowth of bacteria from either urine or vaginal discharge.

Past Medical History

Hospitalization or history of serious illness

Gives an insight into patient's past health. Concurrent illnesses may affect your treatment of the present problem (e.g. aspirin is contraindicated if the patient is on anticoagulants).

Diabetes mellitus

Glycosuria associated with diabetes favors growth of monilia. In diabetes there is an increased glycogen content in vaginal epithelium. Monilial infections often occur when the blood glucose level is over 250 mg./100 ml.

History of venereal disease or vaginitis

A history of similar problems may be useful in diagnosis of the present complaint. However, do not be too quick to ascribe the present problem to venereal disease just because of the history.

Allergies

Penicillin
Tetracycline
Sulfa

Will affect choice of treatment.

OBJECTIVE DATA:

Vital signs

Fever may be associated with salpingitis, pelvic abscess, gonococcemia or secondarily infected herpes progenitalis. The other signs are not as helpful but should be done as part of the general exam.

Pelvic Exam

Inflammation of Bartholin's and Skene's glands

Acute inflammation of a Bartholin's gland is usually secondary to gonorrhea, and is usually unilateral. The infected duct may be surrounded by erythema, and pus can be exuded from the posterior aspect of the labia majora. Chronic Bartholin's cysts are rarely secondary to gonorrhea. Less frequently, this is the site of trichomonal infection.

Sores

In primary syphilis the chancre is the earliest clinical manifestation of disease. It appears at the site of entrance 21-90 days after exposure. Lesions tend to be single and painless, but pain may occur from secondary inflammation or infection. Classically, it is an eroded papule, usually associated with painless inguinal adenopathy. The chancre may persist for 2-6 weeks and heal spontaneously. Lesions of herpes progenitalis are usually vesicular, and are found on the vulva, labia or surrounding skin. Mucosal lesions may appear as yellowish-gray plaques, are very painful and generally heal in 1-2 weeks.

Rashes

The rash associated with secondary syphilis is usually macular with a papulosquamous eruption, especially on the palms of hands and soles of feet. There is a history of exposure to syphilis 2-6 months previously. The rash may be associated with nontender regional adenopathy. The rash associated with gonococcemia is usually papular or petechial, or composed of hemorrhagic pustules most commonly located on the lower extremities.

Venereal warts	Condyloma acuminatum may cause vaginal itching and irritation. Lesions are flesh-colored, cauliflower papules that may occur singularly or in groups.
Redness or swelling of urethra	Urethritis may be secondary to gonorrhea or other causative organisms, especially after local trauma, e.g. frequent intercourse.
Vaginal lesions	These may appear in the form of a chancre, herpes or condyloma acuminatum.
Injection of vaginal mucosa	Hyperemia and petechiae may occur in presence of trichomonads or any other causative organisms. Pallor of vaginal mucosa is usually secondary to atrophic changes.
Character of discharge	See previous description under Subjective Rationale.
Foul odor	See Subjective Rationale.
Cervical erosion	Any vaginal infection may cause loss of the epithelial covering of the cervix due to irritation.
Discharge from cervical os	Implies infection is in uterus or fallopian tubes.
Cervical tenderness	Movement of infected cervix and uterus causes traction on the inflamed tubes in salpingitis, with resultant pain; there may also be some peritoneal inflammation. Salpingitis is usually caused by gonorrhea.
Uterine masses	May be secondary to fibroids, pregnancy or tumor.

Adnexal masses

Can result from inflammatory processes leading to acute swelling or chronic fibrosis. Adnexal fullness may also result from ectopic pregnancy.

Adnexal tenderness

May be indicative of salpingitis, pelvic abscess, ectopic pregnancy, ovarian cyst or tumor.

Inguinal adenopathy

Indicative of local reaction to infection. Tenderness is more common with acute inflammatory processes.

Abdominal Exam

Tenderness on abdominal exam as well as pelvic exam may aid in localization of cause of problem. See Abdominal Pain Protocol.

Lab Data
CBC

Leukocytosis may be present in salpingitis, pelvic abscess, gonococcemia.

ESR (Erythrocyte Sedimentation Rate)

Elevation of ESR above 15 mm. per hour Westergren is usually present in salpingitis. The ESR is also elevated in pregnancy and systemic illnesses.

Wet prep

A sample of vaginal discharge, suspended in a drop of normal saline, is examined microscopically. The presence of numerous motile, flagellate organisms slightly larger than a white blood cell is characteristic of trichomoniasis.

KOH prep

10-40 % potassium hydroxide dissolves debris and lyses cells in the sample of vaginal discharge, thus making hyphae more visible.

Monilia may be seen either as mycelia, which are fiber-like structures with branches (hyphae) or Candida conidia (budding cells).

Gravindex

In the presence of adnexal masses or tenderness, or abdominal pain and history of late or missed periods, the gravindex may help determine if the patient is pregnant. Possibility of tubal pregnancy must be considered in this circumstance.

Urinalysis

See Dysuria Protocol.

ASSESSMENT AND THERAPY:

The four most common types of vaginitis are due to monilia, trichomonas, gonococcus and hemophilus vaginalis. Included in this discussion are the causative organisms, the clinical signs and symptoms, diagnostic and therapeutic measures.

Monilia

Moniliasis is caused by the fungus *C. albicans*. The causative organism may consist of two parts: (1) mycelia, which are long filamentous structures that are usually branched, or (2) conidia, which are buds, usually the size of leukocytes, but which may vary considerably in size.

Most women usually present with the complaint of vaginal or vulvar itching in the presence or absence of vaginal discharge. Associated symptoms include dysuria, frequency of urination and dyspareunia.

Moniliasis is more commonly found in patients with diabetes mellitus, those on oral contraceptives or corticosteroids and patients who have recently received broad spectrum antibiotics. Diabetes and oral contraceptives are believed to alter the glycogen content of the vaginal epithelium, thus producing a good medium in which the organism can grow.

Classically, the discharge of moniliasis is thick, white and curd-like. There may be evidence of erythema and excoriation of the skin secondary to scratching. The vaginal introitus may be inflamed and congested, and in severe cases the inflammation may extend as far as the thighs.

Diagnosis can be made by spreading a small amount of the discharge on a slide and adding a drop of 10-40 % potassium hydroxide (wet prep).

The organism may appear either in the mycelia stage or in the budding cell stage. At times, the diagnosis cannot be made by the wet prep. However, Candida will often grow on Thayer-Martin medium or Nickerson medium, even though the wet prep is negative.

The most common therapeutic agent used is nystatin (Mycostatin) vaginal suppositories.

Trichomonal vaginitis

The causative organism of trichomonal vaginitis is a protozoan, *T.*

vaginalis. Trichomoniasis affects both sexes, and since it is transmitted by sexual intercourse it is most commonly seen during the years of sexual activity. Trichomoniasis may co-exist with moniliasis or gonorrhea.

Trichomonads are highly motile cells, slightly larger than leukocytes but smaller than epithelial cells. The anterior portion has a protruding flagella. Diagnosis is made by suspending a drop of the vaginal discharge in several drops of normal saline and looking for motile forms under the microscope.

The presenting symptom is usually a heavy, greenish-yellow, foul-smelling vaginal discharge. Associated symptoms include vulvar soreness, itching and dyspareunia. Some women may be asymptomatic, whereas the male is rarely symptomatic. Trichomoniasis occurs more frequently in pregnancy and shortly after the menstrual cycle. It is rarely found in virgins.

On the physical exam, the external genitalia may be hyperemic or edematous. The vaginal mucosa may be fiery red with petechiae. In severe infections, there may be blood-tinged discharge from petechial oozing. There may or may not be cervical erosion. Even if cervical erosion is present, the inflammation is not usually found past the cervical os.

The most commonly prescribed treatment is metronidazole (Flagyl) oral tablets, sometimes in conjunction with Flagyl vaginal suppositories. Controversy exists regarding the concurrent treatment of the sexual partner. Since some males can be asymptomatic carriers by harboring the organism in the prepuce or prostatic gland, some believe the regular male partner should also be treated.

Some side effects commonly attributed to Flagyl are nausea, vomiting, intolerance to alcohol and occasionally headaches and dizziness. It is not recommended for administration during the first trimester of pregnancy or to nursing mothers.

Gonorrhea

Gonorrhea is the most commonly reported communicable disease in the United States. The causative organism is *N. gonorrhoeae*. The incubation period is 3-5 days. Most frequent sites of infection are the urethra, anus, cervix, pharynx and the conjunctiva. Some complications seen in the female include urethritis, salpingitis, bartholinitis. Systemic infections include arthritis, meningitis and endocarditis. One of the organism's chief characteristics is that it may remain viable for long periods of time without producing symptomatology.

Infection may occur in several forms. In uncomplicated cases, the female may present with dysuria, frequency and increased vaginal discharge. Frequently there is involvement of the Skene's and Bartholin's glands. In a small percentage of females the infection progresses to involvement, not only of the cervix but also of the fallopian tubes. These patients may present with lower abdominal cramping, fever and dysmenorrhea. Salpingitis may show an increased incidence within the 10 days after the menstrual cycle begins. In patients with pelvic inflammatory disease secondary to gonococcal infection, pain on cervical motion and uterine and adnexal tenderness is usually present, accompanied by an elevation in the ESR. If the infection progresses, adnexal fullness or masses secondary to fibrosis or abscess may occur.

Disseminated gonococcal infections usually have the following symptoms: fever, chills, abdominal pain, monoarticular arthralgias or arthritis without a history of trauma, tenosynovitis and papular, pustular skin eruptions usually on the lower extremities.

Until 5-7 years ago, the most common diagnostic measure was a gram stain of the discharge which showed gram-negative intracellular diplococci. The method is 30-40 % less sensitive than the culture method and may yield false positives. The culture medium of choice is Thayer-Martin, which contains antibiotics that greatly reduce the overgrowth of contaminating organisms. This eliminates growth of organisms which can be mistaken for *N. gonorrhoeae.*

The most effective site for a screening culture is the cervix. In suspicious cases, a rectal culture should also be obtained because it increases the yield of positive culture by 5 %. If the cultures are negative and there is strong suspicion for gonorrhea, they should be repeated again in several days.

The treatment of choice is procaine penicillin in conjunction with probenecid orally. See current U.S. Public Health Service literature for dose.

In penicillin-allergic individuals, tetracycline or spectinomycin may be used. The patient should be told to return in 1 week for a repeat culture because of a 10-15 % treatment failure rate. There should also be an emphasis on notifying sexual contacts. Sexual intercourse should be avoided until the reculture is performed and the cure verified.

Nonspecific or hemophilus vaginitis

The causative organism is often *H. vaginalis* which is a nonmotile, nonencapsulated bacteria. The organism is sexually transmitted, and is usually most common in the reproductive years. Frequently the patient may be asymptomatic or may complain of mild vaginal discharge. When present, the discharge is usually gray and homogeneous and has a less offensive odor than that of trichomoniasis. Secondary vaginal irritation and erythema is rarely observed because the organism does not invade living tissue. On stained smears, the vaginal discharge shows clue cells (granular-appearing, squamous epithelial cells) containing large amounts of short, gram-negative bacilli.

Diagnosis may be made by the gram stain or by exclusion of trichomonads and moniliads. AVC suppositories or vaginal cream are the therapeutic agents of choice.

Herpes progenitalis

Herpes progenitalis is probably the most common cause of vesiculo-ulcerative disease of the genitalia. It is caused by the herpes simplex type II virus, is usually acquired by sexual contact and has an incubation period of 3-7 days.

The primary lesions appear as indurated papules often with vesicle and ulcer formation. Extensive vulvar involvement produces major patient discomfort usually with dysuria and inguinal lymphadenopathy. Lesions may become secondarily infected.

Recurrences are common and represent exacerbation of the dormant virus rather than reinfection. This recurrent nature of the virus makes it particularly difficult to treat.

There is some question regarding the relationship of herpes progenitalis and subsequent occurrence of cervical carcinoma. Pap smears are recommended on a regular basis (yearly) for women with recurrent herpes infections. Infection during pregnancy, with vaginal delivery, poses a risk of infection to the infant. Cesarean section probably should be performed if the infection is active.

Treatment consists of palliative measures such as warm baths, tannic acid applications (apply moist tea bags) and treatment of concurrent vaginitis.

Ectopic pregnancy

Because of the potential for serious sequelae, ectopic pregnancy should be considered in any woman presenting with vaginal or lower abdominal complaints. Classically, it presents as a triad of anomalous menses, pelvic pain and a tender pelvic mass. It does not present as vaginal discharge alone but the two entities can coexist. Therefore, if the history and exam suggest ectopic pregnancy, gynecologic consultation should be sought immediately.

PLAN:

Gonorrhea culture

To rule out gonorrhea.

VDRL

To rule out concurrent syphilis.

Blood glucose

Fasting blood sugar with 2 hour postprandial in persons with recurrent moniliasis to rule out diabetes.

Admit

Suspected ectopic pregnancy, gonococcemia, tubo-ovarian abscess.

Gynecology consult

For diagnostic problems and discharge refractory to the usual modes of therapy.

Patient education
Return if not improved

Seems self-explanatory but the patient should be encouraged to do so.

Call for results of
culture and return for
reculture

If gonorrhea culture is positive, the patient must be informed so she can notify her sexual contacts. Reculture is necessary as there is a 10 % treatment failure rate.

Proper use of
suppositories

The patient should lie down for about ½ hour after inserting them. Bedtime is the most convenient hour for the evening dose.

BIBLIOGRAPHY

Criswell, Sue B., Charles L. Ladwig, and Herman L. Gardner, et al.: "Haemophilus Vaginalis: Vaginitis by Inoculation from Culture," *Obstetrics and Gynecology,* vol. 33, no. 2, February 1969.

Fitzpatrick, Thomas B., Kenneth A. Arndt, and Wallace H. Clark, Jr., et al.: *Dermatology in General Medical Practice,* New York: McGraw Hill, pp. 1957-1961, 1971.

Greenhill, J. P.: *Office Gynecology,* Chicago: Year Book Medical Publishers, pp. 80-93, 1971.

McCann, J., and J. Sidney: "Comparison of Direct Microscopy and Culture in the Diagnosis of Trichomoniasis," *British Journal of Venereal Disease,* vol. 50, pp. 450-452, 1974.

McKinnon, Donald A., and Eleanor B. Rodgerson: "A New Treatment for Yeast Vaginitis," *Obstetrics and Gynecology,* vol. 42, no. 3, pp. 460-464, September 1973.

Oriel, J. D., Betty M. Partridge, and Maire J. Dinny, et al.: "Genital Yeast Infections," *British Medical Journal,* pp. 761-763, December 30, 1972.

Schroeter, Arnold L., and James B. Lucas: "Gonorrhea—Diagnosis and Treatment," *Obstetrics and Gynecology,* pp. 274-284, vol. 39, February 1972.

Watt, Leslie: "Trichomoniasis," *The Practitioner,* vol. 195, pp. 613-619, November 1965.

Wintrobe, Maxwell M., et al. (eds.): *Harrison's Principles of Internal Medicine,* New York: McGraw Hill, pp. 788-792, 1974.

NOTES

NOTES

Chronic
disease
protocols

INTRODUCTION TO CHRONIC DISEASE PROTOCOLS

This section of the book consists of five chronic disease protocols which should be useful in caring for patients with these common, long-term conditions. Several of these protocols are in use in our setting and have already undergone several revisions. Other protocols have not been tested formally.

The use of each of the protocols assumes two things:

1. The diagnosis is established.
2. The protocol will be modified as necessary to recognize concurrent health problems.

The worksheets in these protocols are somewhat different from those described in the acute problem protocols. The Subjective Data part of the worksheet is similar to the acute problem protocols and a new worksheet can be used for each visit. The Objective Data part of the protocol is in the form of a flow sheet that can be kept separately in the patient's chart. We have found it useful to keep the flow sheet next to the patient's problem list. The flow sheet contains two types of information. Some of the data, such as medication, dosage and laboratory results, can be entered directly on the flow sheet. Other data, such as physical exam findings and urinalysis results, cannot be recorded in such a small space and should be entered in the body of the chart (progress note). The flow sheet in this instance will provide an indication of the parameters being followed and the date that a given procedure has been performed.

The Assessment will also differ from the acute problem protocols.

Since the disease is presumably known, the assessment will consist of a description of the patient's present status and his response to the management regime. The Plan and Patient Education sections are perhaps more important with chronic diseases than with acute self-limited problems, many of which may resolve on their own. Management of a chronic disease requires a long-term plan and close patient involvement and cooperation.

These protocols should help establish a consistent data base for nurse practitioner/physician teams. The flow sheet displays data in an organized fashion, and provides a quick overview of the patient's course. The protocols should be adopted, either wholly or in part, depending upon your particular clinic situation and need.

Chapter 14

Chronic obstructive pulmonary disease

CHRONIC OBSTRUCTIVE PULMONARY DISEASE PROTOCOL

Chronic Obstructive Pulmonary Disease (COPD) is a general classification used to encompass chronic bronchitis, emphysema and asthma with its associated bronchitis. These diseases all interfere with the normal process of breathing by obstructing the flow of air in and out of the lungs. Chronic cough, expectoration and shortness of breath, particularly on exertion, are symptoms common to each component of this disease. Management goals for the patient with COPD include:

1. Removal of inciting causes of disease
    a. Irritants (air pollution, industrial pollutants, inhalants, cigarette smoking)
    b. Repeated respiratory infections
2. Treatment of reversible factors of disease
    a. Bronchospasm
    b. Bronchomucosal edema
    c. Airway obstruction due to increased secretions
3. Early recognition and treatment of complications
    a. Bronchial infections/pneumonia
    b. Cor pulmonale
    c. Congestive heart failure
    d. Respiratory failure
4. Patient education and retraining for maximum use of remaining pulmonary function
    a. Instruct patient concerning his disease in lay terms

    b. Explain, and assist patient in complying with, medical manage-
       ment program
       1. Medication
       2. Bronchial hygiene
       3. Breathing retraining
       4. Graded exercise program
5. Improvement of the quality of life as well as extension of life

CHRONIC OBSTRUCTIVE PULMONARY DISEASE WORKSHEET

Positive response indicates management *problem* (describe all positive responses):

Yes   *No*

____ ____ Dyspnea: _____

____ ____ Cough: _____

____ ____ Sputum: _____

____ ____ Smoking:

        Number of cigarettes: _____

        Other: _____

Positive response indicates management *compliance:*

Yes   *No*

____ ____ Taking medications as ordered

____ ____ Bronchial hygiene:

        Number of times/day: _____

        Bronchodilator: _____

        Steam: _____

        Postural drainage: _____

—— —— Graded exercise:

Increased: _____

Decreased: _____

Same: _____

Activity level: _____

SUBJECTIVE RATIONALE:

Dyspnea

Although there is a direct relationship between dyspnea and the amount of lung damage, intermittent infection or irritation can increase the patient's breathlessness. The increase in sputum and bronchospasm can temporarily increase airway obstruction and decrease ventilation.

Cough

A reflex action to clear an irritant, such as particulate foreign bodies or excess secretions, from the bronchial tree. This reflex is of utmost importance to the patient with COPD to aid in maintenance of open airways and to decrease hypoventilation.

Sputum

Production of excess secretions is characterized by the expectoration of whitish sputum. If there is an increase in amount of sputum, there is an increase in bronchial irritation. Should the sputum change from white to yellow or green, it is indicative of respiratory infection. All infections demand immediate treatment since patients with COPD already have compromised pulmonary function and further

CHRONIC OBSTRUCTIVE PULMONARY DISEASE FLOW SHEET

Name
I.D. No.
Age

Dates							
BP/P							
Weight							
Edema							
Chest Exam							
CXR							
EKG							
FEV$_1$/FVC							
pH							

Physical Exam

X-Ray Exam Data

Lab and	pO$_2$/pCO$_2$						
	BUN/K						
	Hct/Hgb						
	Sputum Culture						
Medications	Medication						
Health Maintenance	Complete P.E.						
	Flu Vaccine						

embarrassment can lead to respiratory failure.

Smoking

An irritant to the bronchial tree which leads to increased secretions, decreased ciliary action and increased airway obstruction.

Compliance with Management Modalities

Assess the patient's understanding of his disease, of the prescribed treatment program and the effectiveness of the treatment program.

Medication
Bronchial hygiene

Can decrease bronchospasm, bronchomucosal edema and clear airways, thereby increasing pulmonary function.

Graded exercise

While this will not actually increase pulmonary function, the general improved condition of the patient can lead to a higher level of activity and an improved quality of life.

Activity level

Describe what the patient is able to do. Description provides a baseline for comparison over time.

OBJECTIVE RATIONALE:
Physical Exam
Blood pressure

Monitor every visit. Elevated pCO_2 can cause a slight elevation of systemic blood pressure, but in patients with unrelieved alveolar hypoventilation, severe CO_2 narcosis has been followed by a fall in systemic blood pressure. With changes in blood pressure, drug side effects should be considered. See also chapter on hypertension.

Pulse

When viewed with other findings, an increase in pulse rate could indicate an acute respiratory infection, congestive heart failure or drug toxicity. Monitor every visit.

Weight

A state of good nutrition is closely related to activity level in patients with COPD. Although obesity is not desirable, it is felt by some authorities that a person with beginning emphysema should never be encouraged to lose weight, since many patients date symptoms of respiratory decompensation from a period of weight loss. It is thought that fat within the abdomen facilitates expiration by maintaining pressure on the diaphragm. Concomitant with weight loss and associated decreased muscular strength, the patient tends to become more short of breath while eating and so eats less and loses more weight. To combat this vicious cycle, numerous small feedings may become necessary to maintain an adequate caloric intake. It is also known, but not clearly understood, that patients with COPD have a higher incidence of peptic ulcer disease. Therefore, frequent feedings may be important to help prevent ulcer disease.

A rapid increase in weight may herald fluid retention and impending heart failure even before subcutaneous edema is evident. Monitor every visit.

Edema

In heart failure, tissue edema occurs because of an upset in the normal balance of capillary filtering and reabsorptive forces. For edema to accumulate, capillary pressures must be sufficiently high to force fluid into the tissues. At the same time, salt and water retention by the kidney occurs to replace the fluid that has left the circulation. If unchecked, persistent pitting edema of lower limbs will occur, and systemic venous congestion becomes evident, i.e. distended neck veins, enlarged and tender liver, ascites. Monitor every visit.

Chest exam
Inspection

The overexpanded lungs of patients with COPD can give an increased AP diameter of the chest and a decrease in the overall expansion. The patient may be observed leaning forward, propped on elbows in an effort to more fully expand the chest by elevation of the clavicles and use of the accessory muscles of respiration, i.e. retraction of the intercostal muscles, use of the sternocleidomastoid muscles. Respiratory rate may be increased and the depth of respirations shallow, with a marked increase in the expiratory phase. Central cyanosis may be observed in patients with a low oxygen tension, while the polycythemic patient may exhibit peripheral cyanosis with normal oxygen tension.

Palpation

Decreased expansion of the chest wall.

Percussion

Hyperresonant percussive note.

Auscultation

Diminished breath sounds, fine rales at lung bases, wheezes and rhonchi which often clear with coughing. Distant heart sounds. Monitor each visit to establish a base line for individual patients. Only in this way will it be possible to assess significant changes.

Lab and X-Ray Exam Data
Chest x-ray exam

In COPD, the chest x-ray exam can reveal an increased radiolucency of the lung fields, a decrease in the peripheral vasculature and low, flat diaphragms (limited excursion on fluoroscopy). The emphysematous patient will show a vertical heart position unless there is associated heart disease which leads to cardiac enlargement (cor pulmonale, congestive heart failure). Monitor yearly or when indicated by symptomatology.

Electrocardiogram

Monitor yearly or when indicated as in cor pulmonale, congestive heart failure or arrhythmias.

Pulmonary function tests

COPD is characterized by a slowing down of the expiratory phase of respiration which can be easily calculated from simple spirometry. When the FEV_1 (forced expiratory volume at one second) is divided by the FVC (forced vital capacity) and equals less than 75 %, airway obstruction is said to exist.

Monitor as indicated by increased symptomatology when increased airway obstruction is suspected; to verify bronchodilator effect of medication; yearly for natural progression of disease.

353

Arterial blood gases

Hypoventilation present in COPD gradually leads to hypoxemia (a decrease in pO_2) and hypercapnia (an increase in pCO_2) to which the patient can adapt. However, any insult which increases airway obstruction or reduces respiratory drive further compromises ventilation and can throw the patient into acute respiratory failure. Whenever there is the suspicion of altered ventilation, arterial blood gases should be drawn. Respiratory failure has been defined as pO_2 below 50 mm. Hg (O_2 saturation below 85 %) or pCO_2 above 50 mm. Hg. These numbers must be considered along with other subjective and objective parameters. Monitor yearly when the patient is stable, to obtain a baseline for comparative studies.

Normal	At Sea Level	5,000 Feet Above Sea Level
pH	7.35-7.45	7.35-7.45
pCO_2	35-40 mm. Hg	34-38 mm. Hg
pO_2	85-95 mm. Hg	65-75 mm. Hg

BUN/K+

Follow in patients on diuretic therapy with potassium depletion and the need for replacement therapy. Consider the side effects of digitalis intoxication if hypokalemia is present and the patient is on a digitalis preparation. Monitor every month x 3 when the diuretic is started, then every 6 months if stable.

Hct/Hgb

Elevated: Polycythemia occurs in the hypoxic patient as compensatory reflexes attempt to increase available oxygen to the tissues.

Since, in COPD, hypoxia is due to inadequate gas exchange in the lungs, increasing the red blood count does not correct the deficit. In fact, with the increased viscosity of the blood, coupled with the circulatory burden present as a result of the primary disease, there may be a decrease in the amount of oxygen delivered to the tissues. Phlebotomy may be indicated in patients with a Hct over 65-70 %. Continuous low flow O_2 which maintains a pO_2 of 60 mm. Hg can prevent secondary erythrocytosis.

Decreased: Investigate possible blood loss, particularly by way of the gastrointestinal tract. High incidence of peptic ulcer disease is associated with COPD. Consider the possible increased risk in patients on steroids.

Monitor yearly or as indicated by symptomatology.

Sputum culture

Do whenever a respiratory infection is present which does not improve with 7 days of broad spectrum antibiotic therapy.

Medications

Listing these on flow sheet allows care-giver to correlate subjective and objective findings with management regime.

Health Maintenance

Complete physical exam yearly for general health maintenance.

Flu vaccine

Should be given yearly on a prophylactic basis.

ASSESSMENT: Make a statement concerning the
                                status or progress of the patient,
                                compliance with and effectiveness
                                of current therapy, presence of
                                coexisting problems or complica-
                                tions.

PLAN:
  Diagnostic   Order tests for regular follow-up or
                                as indicated by coexisting problems
                                or suspected complications.

  Therapeutic   Maintain or make alterations in line
                                with current assessment.

The following classifications of drugs commonly are used in the treatment of patients with COPD:

Medication	Action	Side Effects
Bronchodilators oral, rectal, inhaled	Relieve broncho-spasm, broncho-mucosal edema and aid in bronchial hygiene	Most preparations exhibit sympathomimetic effects such as nervousness, insomnia, palpitations, nausea, headaches. The xanthines cause gastrointestinal irritation, and the ephedrine group is known to lead to urinary hesitancy and retention.
Antibiotics	Treat acute respiratory infections. Prophylactic maintenance.	Gastric irritation, nausea, vomiting, diarrhea, skin rash, sore mouth/tongue.
Diuretics	Management of edema with resultant improvement in pulmonary gas exchange.	Anorexia, nausea, vomiting, diarrhea, constipation, headaches, orthostatic hypotension, electrolyte imbalance.

Medication	Action	Side Effects
Potassium supplements	Replace potassium loss from diuretic therapy.	Insufficient replacement results in paresthesias of extremities, mental confusion, listlessness, drop in blood pressure, cardiac arrhythmias.
Digitalis preparations	Increase the mechanical efficiency of heart by increasing the force of systolic contraction, to treat impending heart failure and relieve existing heart failure.	Anorexia, nausea, vomiting, visual disturbances, mental confusion, cardiac arrhythmias (particularly in acute respiratory failure due to low pO_2).
Steroids	Anti-inflammatory properties diminish swelling and narrowing of airways.	Sodium, fluid retention, congestive heart failure, hypokalemia, gastrointestinal irritation with possible peptic ulcer disease, hypertension.
Oxygen	Combat hypoxemia on intermittent or continuous basis.	In patients who have adapted to high levels of pCO_2, the main respiratory stimulus is hypoxemia. If high concentrations of O_2 are administered, this stimulus can be removed and lead to further hypoventilation.

The initiation of any program of home oxygen therapy should only come about as the result of collaboration with the supervising physician. A specific indication for the use of oxygen is the patient with cor pul-

Medication	Action	Side Effects

monale who demonstrates a reversibility of this condition when oxygen is administered. There are many variables to be considered in most cases before home oxygen is ordered, e.g. altitude at which the patient lives, blood gases (awake and asleep), activity level (adaptation to disease process), decreased ease of mobility, cost vs. overall benefit.

Patient education

To be guided by subjective data: patient compliance with treatment plan.

To be guided by objective data: effectiveness of treatment plan.

Should include periodic review of treatment modalities.

BIBLIOGRAPHY

Beeson, Paul B., and Walsh McDermott: *Cecil–Loeb Textbook of Medicine,* Philadelphia: Saunders, 1975.

Belinkoff, Stanton: *Emphysema and Chronic Bronchitis,* Boston: Little, Brown, 1971.

Hinshaw, H. Corwin, and Henry L. Garland: *Diseases of the Chest,* Philadelphia: Saunders, 1963.

Hudak, Carolyn M., Barbara M. Gallo, and Thelma Lohr: *Critical Care Nursing,* Philadelphia: Lippincott, 1973.

Nett, Louise M., and Thomas L. Petty, "Effective Treatment for Emphysema and Chronic Bronchitis," *Journal of Rehabilitation,* pp. 10-12, 53-56, September-October 1967.

Petty, Thomas L., and Louise M. Nett: *For Those Who Live and Breathe with Emphysema and Chronic Bronchitis,* Springfield, Illinois: Charles C Thomas, 1967.

Walker, H. Kenneth, Willis J. Hurst, and Mary F. Woody (eds.): *Applying the Problem Oriented System,* New York: MedCom, 1973.

NOTES

NOTES

Chapter 15

Diabetes
mellitus

DIABETES MELLITUS PROTOCOL

Diabetes mellitus (DM) is a chronic, systemic disease characterized by the inability of the pancreatic beta cells to produce sufficient, if any, insulin. The fundamental defects to which many of the clinical symptoms can be traced are: 1) a reduced entry or transport of glucose from the blood to the cells/tissues of the body and, 2) an increased liberation of glucose into the circulating blood from the liver. There is, therefore, an extracellular glucose excess and an intracellular glucose deficiency, a situation which has been called "starvation in the midst of plenty."

Predisposition to diabetes mellitus is inherited. There is much controversy regarding this inheritance, with some researchers claiming it resembles that of an autosomal recessive trait, while others cite multifactorial inheritance. Incidence of the disease has been noted as occurring in 2 % of the child population and 10 % of the adult population. Obesity, increasing age and number of pregnancies are also thought to be contributory factors.

Categories of Diabetes Mellitus:

There are two major categories of diabetes mellitus: 1) juvenile diabetes and, 2) adult onset diabetes.

Juvenile Onset (growth onset)

This type has its onset in childhood or adolescence, is often severe and is characterized by episodes of hyperglycemia and hypoglycemia. While the term "brittle" is often associated with juvenile onset diabetes, one must be wary of generalization, since adult onset diabetics are occasionally brittle. Etiology stems from the inability of the pancreatic beta cells to produce insulin.

In managing the adult with diabetes mellitus, the duration of the disease is significant. It is unusual to detect clinical evidence of vascular lesions during the first ten years of the disease. The adult patient with juvenile onset diabetes is more likely to show evidence of complications as the result of chronic long term changes of small and large vessels.

Adult Onset Diabetes

Diabetes developing after age 35 is generally mild, and ketoacidosis is rare. This condition is often the result of a delayed release of endogenous insulin in relation to carbohydrate challenge. However, some adult onset patients may have a sub-normal capacity for insulin synthesis and release.

COMPLICATIONS:

Small Vessel Changes (Microangiopathy)

Pathophysiology: There is a basic deposition of glycoprotein in the basement membranes of arterioles, causing thickening of the vessel wall, narrowing of the lumen and loss of elasticity. The nature of pathology for the individual patient will depend on the organs in which these arteriolar changes take place. Organs which are most readily affected are the eye (exhibited as retinopathy, glaucoma, cataract formation and extraocular palsies) and the kidney (diabetic glomerulosclerosis, arteriolar nephrosclerosis and pyelonephritis).

Large Vessel Changes

Pathophysiology: These changes stem from increased serum cholesterol and triglycerides resulting in atherosclerosis of large vessels. Symptoms arise from insufficient blood supply to the central nervous system, brain, lower extremities and especially the heart (coronary arteries).

DIABETES MELLITUS WORKSHEET

Positive response and/or change may indicate management *problem* (describe all positive responses):

SYMPTOMS ARISING FROM INSUFFICIENT INSULIN:

Yes   No

____ ____ Hyperglycemic reactions (dry skin, flushed face, thirst, nausea, vomiting, abdominal pain, drowsiness, rapid pulse, blurred vision, constipation and deep Kussmaul respirations imply ketoacidosis and necessitate immediate treatment): _____

——— ——— Polyuria/nocturia:_____

——— ——— Glycosuria (positive dipstick readings): _____

——— ——— Polydipsia:_____

——— ——— Polyphagia: _____

——— ——— Weight loss (involuntary):_____

——— ——— Fatigue: _____

SYMPTOMS ARISING FROM EXCESSIVE INSULIN:
Yes   *No*

——— ——— Hypoglycemic reactions (periods of nervousness, fatigue, headache, hunger, tremor, faintness, diplopia, pallor,

sweating, irrational behavior, etc.): _____

_____

SYMPTOMS OR COMPLAINTS ARISING FROM CHRONIC COMPLICATIONS:
Yes   *No*

——— ——— Skin:

_____Boils–pruritus, especially vulvar: _____

_____Ulcers:_____

_____Rash: _____

——— ——— Eyes:

_____Decreased vision/visual changes: _____

_____Specks, cobwebs, floaters in visual fields: _____

_____Problem moving eyes: _____

Chronic Disease Protocols

___ ___ Mouth:

     _____Dental caries: _____

     _____Sore/inflamed gums: _____

___ ___ Central nervous system:

     _____Numbness, tingling, burning pain in extremities,

     muscle cramps:_____

___ ___ Cardiovascular:

     _____Chest pain, shortness of breath: _____

     _____Color changes, temperature changes, pain in

     extremities: _____

     _____Intolerance to cold in hands/feet: _____

___ ___ Gastrointestinal:

     _____Diarrhea—especially nocturnal, early AM: _____

     _____

___ ___ Genitourinary:

     _____Impotence:_____

     _____Flank pain, edema: _____

     _____Perineal itching/vaginal discharge:_____

___ ___ Psychosocial:

     _____Is there anything bothering patient,

     such as problems at home, etc.?:_____

_____ _____ Other chronic diseases: _____

_____ _____ Acute infections: _____

_____ _____ Medications: _____

_____

_____

SUBJECTIVE RATIONALE:
*Symptoms Arising from
Insufficient Insulin*
    Etiology

Causes include omission of insulin injection, dietary indiscretions (not following the prescribed diet, especially ingestion of alcoholic and carbohydrate-containing products), inadequate amount of prescribed insulin, presence of intercurrent illness or emotional stress.

    Ketoacidosis

In the face of insufficient or no insulin there exists an inability of glucose transport from the blood to the body's cells and organ tissues. Blood glucose is high and:

1. Absence of insulin activates hormone sensitive lipase which

2. Converts body fat to free fatty acids in the blood which

3. Are transported to the liver and converted into acetyl coenzyme A. Some of this can act as a source of body energy, but usually too great an amount is made so it is transported back to the liver and

DIABETES MELLITUS FLOW SHEET

Name
I.D. No.
Age

Dates								
Weight								
B/P								
Eyes/Fundi								
Pinpoint Test								
Skin								
Cardiac								
Feet Edema/lesions								
Pulses								
Neuropathy								
Blood Glucose								
Na	Cl								
K	CO_2								
BUN/Creat.								

Physical Examination

		Cholesterol/ Triglycerides							
Lab Data		24 hr. glucose							
		24 hr. protein							
		Creat. Cl.							
	Urine	Glucose							
		Prot.							
		Acetone							
Medications		Oral agents							
		Insulin							
Health Maintenance		Diet							
		CBC/EKG							
		Chest x-ray							
		Pap/Rectal Exam/Full P.E.							
		M.D. Visit							

4. Converted to acetoacetic acid. Again, a certain amount can be used for energy but the excess is converted to

5. Hydroxybutyric acid and acetone. Acetoacetic acid, hydroxybutyric acid and acetone are ketone bodies, increased levels of which produce a ketoacidotic state.

Polyuria/nocturia

When a heavy solute load exists in the blood (hyperglycemia) the resultant increase in osmotic pressure draws water out of the tissues. This increased load of water and glucose passes through the glomerulus of the kidney into the urine.

Glycosuria

The capacity of the kidney to reabsorb glucose is limited to 160 mg. %, the usual renal threshold. In the presence of high blood glucose levels, when the glomerular filtrate passes through the kidney, only a *fixed* amount can be reabsorbed; the remainder will spill into the urine. This sign is of limited value in the elderly diabetic, who as a result of normal aging has reduced kidney function and often exhibits a high renal threshold.

Polydipsia

There are two causes: 1) patient is losing large amounts of water secondary to polyuria, 2) increased blood glucose, decreased blood volume and increased blood osmotic pressure all stimulate the thirst mechanism in the brain.

Polyphagia

The hypothalamus, in addition to the thirst center, has an appetite and satiety center. The appetite center is tonically active and is depressed by the satiety center which has as its function the monitoring of glucose in the surrounding areas. If cell glucose is low, the satiety center does not depress the active state of the appetite center and the patient experiences constant hunger.

Weight loss (involuntary)

Since there is inadequate or no glucose available for energy (due to inability to transport glucose into cells with lack of insulin), the body utilizes both fat (as previously described) and protein as secondary sources of energy. The results of protein breakdown, in addition to weight loss, are negative nitrogen balance, decreased antibodies and WBC count. (This is thought to play a significant role in the diabetic's susceptibility to infections.)

Fatigue

Decreased transport of glucose into the cells decreases the available fuel for body energy with resulting fatigue.

Symptoms Arising from Excessive Insulin
Etiology

Hypoglycemia is an ever-present possibility in the patient who takes insulin or oral hypoglycemic agents. Situations which predispose to hypoglycemia ("insulin reaction") include a delay in or omission of a meal, an increase in the amount of exercise taken, periods of emotional stress or an improvement in the patient's glucose tolerance. Errors in the measurement of insulin resulting in excessive dosage can also be responsible.

Hypoglycemic reactions	Low blood glucose levels produce symptoms referable to the central nervous system and autonomic nervous system.
Central nervous system symptoms	In the presence of low blood glucose levels (less than 50 mg./100 ml. blood), behavior changes such as mental confusion, disorientation, aimless hyperactivity, hallucinations, convulsions and coma occur.
Autonomic nervous system symptoms	In response to decreased blood glucose there is a massive outpouring of catecholamines with resultant tachycardia and activation of arousal centers causing anxiety, diaphoresis, pallor and hypotension.

Symptoms or Complaints Arising from Chronic Complications

Skin

Boils	Among complications involving the skin of the diabetic are furuncles and carbuncles. In the normal individual, the skin serves as a storehouse for glycogen. In uncontrolled diabetes and hyperglycemia, the glycogen in the skin is depleted and the glucose content increases, predisposing the skin to infections, especially staphylococcal. There is also evidence that function of polymorphonuclear leukocytes is impaired.
Ulcers	Due to poor circulation secondary to large vessel changes, the tissues in the feet and legs of the diabetic have poor resistance to infection, so that minor trauma and abrasions result in ulcerations.

Rash/lesions

Mycosis (any disease caused by a fungus) may be manifested by development upon the face, scalp and chest of firm, reddish tumors that are painful and have a tendency to spread and ulcerate. Less severe types of fungus infection are also common.

Xanthoma diabeticorum–formation of reddish solid patches, sometimes appearing with yellow spots at top of lesion, and thought to be secondary to lipid deposits.

Necrobiosis lipoidica diabeticorum–a dermatosis characterized by patchy degeneration of the elastic and connective tissue of the skin. Occurs primarily on pre-tibial surfaces and is of cosmetic importance only.

Eyes
Decreased vision/visual changes

Changes are noted to take place: 1) in the retina, which on funduscopic exam are seen as venous microaneurysms, hemorrhages and exudative processes, culminating in the picture of a proliferative retinopathy; 2) in the lens (diabetic cataract) secondary to hyperglycemia, due to conversion of glucose to sorbitol which osmotically draws water into lens.

Hemorrhagic glaucoma may also occur.

Problem of eye movement

Extraocular muscle palsies occur, sometimes preceded by pain on affected side; usually the 3rd or 6th nerve is involved, with the latter being most commonly involved. This is secondary to neuropathy.

Mouth
Dental caries
Sore-inflamed gums

These conditions seem to occur more often in diabetics. If the infection becomes severe (e.g. abscess) it may disrupt diabetic control.

Central Nervous System
Numbness, tingling,
burning sensation
of extremities

Neurological disturbances are common; the two most often implicated are related to dysfunction of the 1) somatic and 2) visceral nerves.

Somatic neuropathy–peripheral neuritis most often presents with pain and paresthesia in the lower extremities. Occasionally, the presenting sign is weakness of the extremity.

Visceral neuropathy–includes those deficiencies in function, such as delayed gastric emptying, bladder involvement, impotence, diarrhea, neurotrophic ulcers and postural or orthostatic hypotension, which are related to the autonomic nervous system and various organs.

Cardiovascular
Chest pain, shortness of breath

Due to large vessel changes. The diabetic is predisposed to pathology affecting coronary arteries resulting in myocardial infarction, angina and congestive heart failure.

Color/temperature changes
Pain in extremities

Secondary to large-vessel disease with resulting ischemia. Intermittent claudication is often the result.

372

Gastrointestinal
Diarrhea

Etiology:

1. Neurogenic/neuropathy.

2. Unknown, probably secondary to No. 1, with resultant bacterial overgrowth in small intestine. Often associated with steatorrhea, which in turn may be a concomitant of pancreatic insufficiency.

Genitourinary
Impotence

This is a manifestation of autonomic visceral damage. In addition, retrograde ejaculation may be present as a complication.

Flank pain/edema

Disease conditions such as pyelonephritis, diabetic glomerulosclerosis, papillary necrosis and arteriolar nephrosclerosis are more prevalent in the diabetic.

Perineal itching
Vaginal discharge

There may be vaginal infection, usually Monilia, due to increased glucose in the vaginal epithelium which provides a good medium for fungal growth.

Psychosocial Problems

The very nature of the chronicity of diabetes and the myriad of possible complications can cause anxiety, depression, dependency and inability to cope with life stresses. This in turn may pose a threat to the individual's self esteem.

Other Chronic Diseases

It is important to manage any other problems, as changes may affect diabetic control.

Acute Infections

May worsen diabetes and even precipitate ketoacidosis. Insulin dosage may have to be temporarily increased.

Other Medications

Antisympathetic drugs, such as propranolol, block action of catecholamines so that the patient may be unaware of an approaching hypoglycemic reaction.

In addition, the thiazides and oral contraceptives may increase blood glucose levels.

OBJECTIVE RATIONALE:

Weight

All patients should be encouraged to maintain normal weight. Weight reduction in the obese adult diabetic patient promotes optimum control and often results in reduction of medication. Monitor every visit.

Blood pressure

Blood pressure should be monitored, given the manifestations of diabetic nephropathy and the increased incidence of generalized atherosclerosis and coronary artery disease if it is uncontrolled. This parameter should be controlled with appropriate medication. Monitor every visit.

Ophthalmoscopy/eye exam

Retinopathy, cataract formation, glaucoma and extraocular muscle palsies are frequent complications in the diabetic patient. The pinpoint eye exam is one of the earliest screening measures to detect macular edema which may be the first sign of retinopathy, before hemorrhages and/or exudates can be noted.

The funduscopic exam may reveal microaneurysms, exudates and the signs of proliferative retinopathy. Monitor every six months and in response to subjective visual changes. The funduscopic exam is no substitute for a yearly complete eye exam by an ophthalmologist which should include tests for visual acuity.

Retinopathy

This is an ominous sign in diabetics, since it carries a significant risk of blindness. Three main stages of retinopathy are stated below:

Stage I–(simple retinopathy)
Physical findings: "red dots" or capillary microaneurysms; possibly some venous dilation.

Stage II–(simple retinopathy)
Physical findings: as enumerated above plus hemorrhages and exudates.

Stage III–(proliferative retinopathy)
Physical findings: all or varying combinations of the above, *plus* subhyaloid and/or vitreous hemorrhage, proliferation of new vessels and fibrous tissue bands. The changes often present first around the disc.

Cataract formation

The two types are metabolic and senile. The metabolic type occurs in young people with severe diabetes, and is related to the degree of control. It is snowflake-like in appearance, and starts in the subcapsular region of the lens. Opacity may increase rapidly but can be temporary and reversible with tighter control of the hyperglycemia in the early stages of this complication.

The senile type is seen in the elderly and does not seem to be more common in the diabetic; it is similar in type to the cataract in the non-diabetic.

Glaucoma

Ophthalmologic exam reveals increased intraocular tension and cupping of disks. This requires immediate ophthalmologic referral.

Skin

Xanthoma diabeticorum, necrobiosis lipoidica diabeticorum, furunculosis, mycosis and pruritus are conditions frequently manifested in the diabetic patient. See Subjective Rationale.

Cardiovascular

Coronary artery disease reportedly accounts for 31 % of all deaths in the United States, as compared to 53 % in a large diabetic population. The duration of the disease, the presence of hyperlipidemia and the coincident presence of diastolic hypertension can be considered contributing factors to this significant problem. Therefore, a cardiac exam should be scheduled every six months. If the patient's history or physical findings give indications of cardiovascular changes, a cardiac exam should be included during that visit. The vascular complications are discussed under examination of the feet.

Examination of the feet	The triad of ischemia, infection and neuropathy promotes the development of major changes in the lower extremities which could lead to decreased healing and possible amputation.
Inspection	Note the presence of ulcers, ingrown toenails, dryness, discoloration, edema and absence of hair growth.
Palpation	Palpate the dorsalis pedis and posterior tibial pulses, record on a numerical scale and note the temperature of extremities.
Other tests	The lower extremities should be tested for deficits in sensory perception:

a. pinprick for pain
b. tuning fork for vibratory sensation
c. manual manipulation of great toe for position sense

Deep tendon reflexes should be elicited. The ankle jerk may be absent or diminished in the long-term diabetic due to concomitant neuropathy.

Fasting blood glucose, 2 hour postprandial glucose	The fasting blood glucose and 2 hour postprandial glucose are monitored frequently to adjust therapy in the uncontrolled diabetic, and every 6 months in the stable diabetic.

Electrolytes
BUN
Creatinine
Cholesterol
Triglycerides
Creatinine clearance
24 hour protein

Given the well-established relationship of diabetes to the development of nephropathy, diabetic glomerulosclerosis, arteriolar nephrosclerosis, pyelonephritis and atherosclerosis, these lab values should be recorded for an initial baseline, then monitored at intervals determined by clinic policy based on patient's objective signs of elevated blood pressure, edema and proteinuria. These parameters should be monitored yearly in a stable diabetic.

Urine glucose, protein and acetone
24 hour urine glucose

These parameters are monitored on each clinic visit to determine the adequacy of control, status of kidney involvement and presence of ketosis.

The 24 hour urine sugar should be between 5-10 gm. for good control.

If unexplained glycosuria and hyperglycemia are present, the practitioner should explore the possibility of intercurrent illness or infection, by doing appropriate systems review or examination.

Medication

See Review of Therapeutic Agents, Table 15-1.

Insulin therapy is currently preferred over oral agents because it is more uniformly effective in controlling hyperglycemia. The results of studies conducted by the University Group Diabetes Program (UGDP), although controversial, suggest that insulin therapy may be safer than the sulfonylureas and the biguanide compounds (DBI) with respect to the mortality rates due to cardiovascular complications. It is unlikely that the use of oral agents will be abandoned; however, it is hoped that the adjunct modes of therapy, adherence to diet and weight reduction, will receive increased attention by the practitioner and the patient. It is noteworthy that only 50 % of all diabetics on sulfonylureas can be controlled by these oral agents beyond a five year period.

Diet

Adherence to a prescribed American Diabetic Association (ADA) diet is of prime importance in management of the disease by the patient. The challenge to the practitioner lies in the crucial aspects of patient education and motivation. 50 % of the diabetic population make *no* attempt to follow a diet.

Health maintenance
CBC

Given the small-vessel disease and the side effect of hemolytic anemia with the sulfonylureas, the CBC should be done yearly.

EKG

Yearly on all diabetic patients over 35. See Objective Rationale under Cardiovascular.

Chest x-ray

Bi-yearly, unless indicated more often on the basis of occupation or environment.

Pap/rectal exam/
full physical exam

Yearly.

TABLE 15-1
REVIEW OF THERAPEUTIC AGENTS

KINDS OF INSULIN

Activity	Type	Onset hrs.	Peak hrs.	Duration hrs.
Rapid-acting	Regular	1-2	2-3	5-7
	Semilente	1-2	4-5	12-16
Intermediate-acting	Isophane (NPH)	2-3	8-10	20-24
	Lente	2-3	8-12	20-24
	Globin (rarely used)			
Long-acting	Protamine Zinc	4-6	12-20	24-36
	Ultralente	5-6	12-28	24-36+

Always provide a 10-15 gm. carbohydrate snack for the peak action period.

ORAL AGENTS

Two groups: 1) Sulfonylureas
           2) Phenformin (DBI)

1) Sulfonylureas—stimulate release of endogenous insulin from pancreatic beta cells.

	Tablet	Daily Dose	Duration	No. Doses/Day
Tolbutamide (Orinase)	500 mg.	0.5-3.0 gm.	6-12 hrs.	2-3
Acetohexamide (Dymelor)	250 mg. 500 mg.	250 mg.- 1500 mg.	12-24 hrs.	1-2
Tolazamide (Tolinase)	100 mg. 250 mg.	100-750 mg.	12-24 hrs.	1-2
Chlorpropamide (Diabinese)	100 mg. 250 mg.	100-500 mg.	24-48 hrs.	1

2) Phenethylbiguanide—mode of action not clearly understood. This agent is thought to increase the rate of anaerobic Phenformin (DBI) glycolysis and facilitate cellular glucose entry.

	Tablet	Daily Dose	Duration	No. Doses/Day
Phenformin (DBI)	25 mg.	50-200 mg.	4-6 hrs.	2-3
DBI-T.D. (Time Delay)	50 mg. capsule	50-200 mg.	8-12 hrs.	1-2

381

TABLE 15-2
PATIENT EDUCATIONAL OBJECTIVES

Pt. Name _____

Pt. Age _____

Duration of Diabetes: _____

Physical, intellectual or language disabilities: _____

Medication—kind: _____
Dosage: _____
How many diabetic classes: _____
When: _____

Diet:
1. Has diabetic and dietary literature
2. Can understand exchanges and calories
3. Can select meals
4. Can convert diet plan to clear and full liquids on sick days

Urine: Is able to:
1. Test urine for sugar—
   —Tes-tape
   —Clinitest—2 gtt.
            5 gtt.
2. Test urine for acetone
3. Keep record of urine tests—(2nd voided spec.)
4. Knows when and how often to test
5. Can correlate urine testing and insulin need

Foot Care:

General Skin Care:

Administration of Insulin:
1. Select correct syringe for correct concentration of insulin
2. Rotate bottle before using

Insulin/Oral Hypoglycemics: Knows:

1. Dosage in units
2. Type of insulin
3. Concentration to use: U. 40, 80, 100
4. Purpose of snack at peak insulin action and at bedtime
5. Use of oral hypoglycemic agents—kind, dosage, side effects

Ketoacidosis (Hyperglycemia): Knows:

1. How to recognize impending ketoacidosis
2. How to avoid ketoacidosis
3. How to treat ketoacidosis

Insulin Reaction (Hypoglycemia): Knows:

1. How to recognize insulin reaction
2. How to avoid reaction
3. How to treat reaction—Knows 10 gm. CHO sources
4. How to use Glucagon Kit—(family member instruction)
5. How to use—Instant Glucose
   or—Neg-React
   or—Reactose

3. Clean rubber stopper on bottle
4. Read syringe
5. Draw up insulin
6. Cleanse skin
7. Insert needle into skin
8. Aspirate for blood
9. Rotate sites for injection (insulin map)

Sick Day Rules:

1. Always take your insulin
2. Test your urine for both sugar and acetone—record results
3. Call your doctor or nurse practitioner
4. Go to bed—keep warm
5. Convert diet to liquids and take liquids every hour
6. NEVER SKIP YOUR INSULIN. You may need extra insulin. If so, take according to the instructions given to you.

Test Education Content By:

1. Paper and pencil tests
2. Oral questions and answer
3. Demonstration/return demonstration

M.D. visit or consultation   Approximately every 3rd visit for the stable diabetic, or as indicated by patient status.

Patient education   A sample outline of patient education objectives is illustrated in Table 15–2.

BIBLIOGRAPHY

Allison, Sarah E.: "A Framework for Nursing Action in a Nurse-Conducted Diabetic Management Clinic," *Journal of Nursing Administration,* pp. 53-61, July-August 1973.

Beland, Irene L.: *Clinical Nursing: Pathophysiological and Psychosocial Approaches,* New York: Macmillan, 1975.

Ganong, W. F.: *Review of Medical Physiology,* Los Altos, California: Lange Medical Publications, 1973.

Goyal, Raj. K. and Howard M. Spiro: "Gastrointestinal Manifestations of Diabetes Mellitus," *Medical Clinics of North America,* vol. 55, pp. 1057-1064, July 1971.

Lilly Research Laboratories: *Diabetes Mellitus,* Indianapolis, Indiana: Eli Lilly and Co., 1967.

Stein, G. H.: "The Use of a Nurse Practitioner in the Management of Patients with Diabetes Mellitus," *Medical Care,* vol. 12, pp. 885-90, October 1974.

Sussman, Karl E., and Stefan S. Fajans (eds.): *Diabetes Mellitus,* vol. III, American Diabetes Association, 1971.

NOTES

NOTES

Chapter 16

Viral
hepatitis

VIRAL HEPATITIS PROTOCOL

To be used for patients with:
Diagnosed Viral Hepatitis.
(This protocol assumes other causes
of jaundice or liver disease have
been ruled out.)

---

*What you can't afford to miss: fulminant hepatitis, acute
hepatic necrosis.*

Although hepatitis is an acute illness, follow-up is relatively long-term
and requires active patient education; therefore, it is included under
chronic illness for purposes of this book.

There are two types of viral hepatitis, HBag positive (serum, type B
or SH) and HBag negative (infectious, type A or IH). These types are
transmissible by similar means, and although HBag positive is often
considered the most "dangerous," treatment and follow-up are the
same. Incubation of HBag positive is 6 weeks to 6 months; HBag negative is 2–6 weeks.

SUBJECTIVE DATA:

A flow sheet containing subjective data can sometimes be useful
(see Table 16-1). However, it leaves little room for comments. The
worksheet described below is somewhat more cumbersome but provides room for additional data.

SUBJECTIVE WORKSHEET
EXPLAIN POSITIVE FINDINGS

Yes　*No*

____　____　Anorexia:

　　　　　　　Diet history: _____

____　____　Fatigue:

　　　　　　　Increasing: _____

　　　　　　　Decreasing: _____

　　　　　　　Activity history: _____

____　____　Arthralgias:

　　　　　　　Location: _____

　　　　　　　Increasing: _____

　　　　　　　Decreasing: _____

____　____　Myalgias:

　　　　　　　Increasing: _____

　　　　　　　Decreasing: _____

____　____　Nausea:

　　　　　　　Increasing: _____

　　　　　　　Decreasing: _____

____　____　Vomiting:

　　　　　　　Number of episodes: _____

　　　　　　　Amount of food retained: _____

---- ---- Diarrhea:

       Increasing: _____

       Decreasing: _____

       Number of stools per day: _____

       Consistency: _____

---- ---- Rash:

       Location: _____

       Increasing: _____

       Decreasing: _____

---- ---- Dark urine:

       Color: _____

       Getting lighter: _____

       Getting darker: _____

---- ---- Light stools:

       Color: _____

       Getting lighter: _____

       Getting darker: _____

---- ---- Pruritus:

       Location: _____

       Increasing: _____

Decreasing: _____

____ ____ Icterus:

Scleral increasing: _____

Scleral decreasing: _____

Skin increasing: _____

Skin decreasing: _____

____ ____ Weight loss:

Amount: _____

____ ____ Easy bruising:

Location: _____

History of trauma: _____

____ ____ Menstrual changes:

Describe: _____

____ ____ Headaches:

Location: _____

Frequency: _____

Duration: _____

Severity: _____

____ ____ Sore throat:

Severity: _____

Increasing: _____

Decreasing: _____

____ ____ Chills:

    Severity: _____

    Duration: _____

    Number of episodes: _____

____ ____ Fever:

    Documented: _____

____ ____ Abdominal pain:

    Location: _____

    Related to: _____

    Severity: _____

    Duration: _____

    Increasing: _____

    Decreasing: _____

____ ____ Drugs:

    Type: _____

    Amount: _____

OBJECTIVE DATA:
See Flow Sheet (Table 16–1)

SUBJECTIVE RATIONALE:

Anorexia

This is an early sign, usually abrupt; the cause is obscure. There may also be a distaste for cigarettes.

TABLE 16-1

HEPATITIS FLOW SHEET*

Name
I.D. No.
Age or birthdate

SUBJECTIVE DATA:

DATE OF VISIT

+ = Present
− = Absent

	By History					
1. Anorexia						
2. Fatigue						
3. Arthralgias						
4. Myalgias						
5. Nausea						
6. Vomiting						

7. Diarrhea				
8. Rash				
9. Dark Urine				
10. Light Stools				
11. Pruritus				
12. Icterus				
13. Weight Loss				
14. Easy Bruising				
15. Menstrual Changes				
16. Headaches				
17. Sore Throat				
18. Chills				
19. Fever				
20. Abdominal Pain				

OBJECTIVE DATA: Vital Signs					
Weight					
Skin: 1. Icterus					
2. Acne					
3. Spider Angiomata					
HEENT: 1. Scleral Icterus					
2. Lymphadenopathy					
Abdomen: 1. Shape					
2. Hepatomegaly					
3. Splenomegaly					
4. Tenderness					
Joints: 1. Erythema					

2. Edema

*This flow sheet is currently being used in the Hepatitis Clinic at Colorado General Hospital. We acknowledge the staff, and particularly Frederic B. Walker, M.D., Assistant Professor of Medicine, University of Colorado, for their efforts in the development and refinement of this tool.

Name
I.D. No.
Age or birthdate

DATE	ASSESSMENTS	*RTC	WORK DISPOSITION

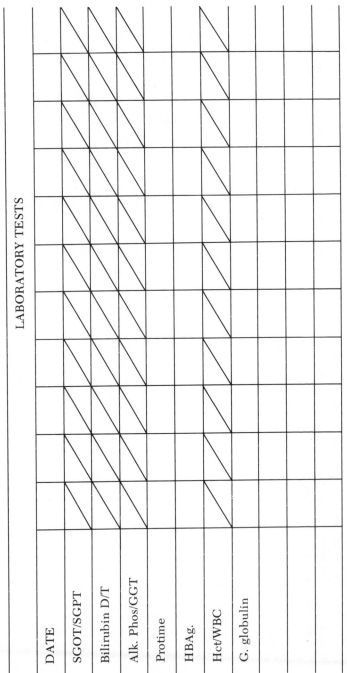

LABORATORY TESTS

DATE										
SGOT/SGPT										
Bilirubin D/T										
Alk. Phos/GGT										
Protime										
HBAg.										
Hct/WBC										
G. globulin										

*RTC = Return to Clinic

Fatigue	Early sign. This can be a prolonged symptom, lasting 6 months to a year.
Arthralgias	Rarely severe enough to incapacitate. This symptom, as well as fatigue, headache, anorexia and fever, may be due to primary liver disease or extra-hepatic effects of the virus.
Myalgias	Same as above.
Nausea	Early sign. The cause is obscure; perhaps due to viral effect.
Vomiting	Antiemetic suppositories may be prescribed. It is a criterion for admission, if so severe that parenteral fluids must be given.
Diarrhea	Not a consistent symptom. In some patients this may be related to malabsorption.
Rash	Cause is obscure. It may be a systemic reaction to the virus or an auto-immune reaction. Acne, if present, may flare, which is a common reaction to body stress. Rash is urticarial, erythematous and maculopapular.
Dark urine	Bilirubin in the urine accounts for the dark color; it is rarely seen in persons without liver disease. In fresh specimens of icteric urine, only conjugated pigments can be detected. They are excreted mainly by glomerular filtration. In viral hepatitis there is poor correlation between conjugated bilirubin in the plasma and that in the urine.

Light stools	Bilirubin is reduced to urobilinogen in the intestine by bacteria. Urobilinogen is normally reabsorbed from the intestine and re-excreted by the liver, giving the stools their normal brown color. In the presence of liver damage, re-excretion is impaired and the stools become light.
Pruritus	Is generalized and caused by retained bile acids which are deposited in the skin. This is not related to the intensity of jaundice. Cholestyramine may be given, although it may produce diarrhea. This drug lowers serum bile acid levels by binding bile salts in the intestine and preventing their reabsorption.
Icterus	Depth of jaundice depends on the concentration of bilirubin in the plasma, on factors that control capillary permeability, diffusion of bilirubin from plasma and binding of bilirubin by the tissues. Jaundice becomes apparent in the sclerae and skin when serum concentration of bilirubin exceeds 2-3 mg./100 ml. Depth of jaundice does not necessarily correlate with severity of hepatitis.
Weight loss	Rapid but rarely severe. It is related to low food ingestion and vomiting.
Easy bruising	Can be a serious sign, and calls for determination of the prothrombin time. Bile salts are essential for the normal digestion and absorption of fat and fat soluble vitamins, one of which is vitamin K. Vitamin K deficiency depresses the synthesis of clotting factors.

Protime

This is the most important test in assessing the degree of liver impairment. By proper use of vitamin K, this test can be made almost completely specific for liver function. Failure of the liver to bring the prothrombin time within normal limits, in the presence of adequate amounts of vitamin K in circulating blood, indicates clinically significant liver impairment. The degree of prothrombin time abnormality closely parallels the degree of liver impairment, and is the most useful diagnostic index in severe liver disease.

H Bag (hepatitis B antigen)

This has been alluded to throughout the protocol. Approximately 1 % of people with HBag positive hepatitis will never "convert" to negative, thereby being in the carrier state. Degree of contagion of carriers is unknown, but is probably low, except by parenteral means.

Hct/WBC

Hemoglobin and hematocrit are normal early in the disease, and usually remain so. White blood cell count may be normal or reduced. If normal, it is usually not repeated during the course of the disease.

Gamma globulin

This is drawn when SGOT/SGPT have not returned to normal in 6-8 weeks. The serum level of gamma globulin, as determined by serum protein electrophoresis, is often markedly elevated in chronic active hepatitis. This presumably reflects the immunologic etiology of the disease. Markedly elevated serum gamma globulin in the presence of liver disease is therefore suggestive, but not diagnostic, of chronic active hepatitis.

ASSESSMENT:

Since all these patients will have diagnosed hepatitis, the assessment is really a description of how the patient is progressing. It is also necessary to be aware of possible complications (see Rationale).

Although most people may be followed safely as outpatients, those with protracted vomiting, and life styles which preclude adequate self-care should be admitted. A prolonged protime (less than 50 %), may call for admission, as this indicates greater liver damage. People over the age of 40 tend to have more difficulty and are often admitted.

Viral hepatitis in the majority of cases is a self-limiting disease. Less than 10-15 % may develop chronic active hepatitis or chronic persistent hepatitis as diagnosed by liver biopsy (see Biopsy Algorithm). These patients will require careful follow-up and possibly steroid therapy. They will not be considered here.

LIVER BIOPSY ALGORITHM*

FOR LIVER DISEASE PRESENTING AS ACUTE SYMPTOMATIC HEPATITIS

Follow at daily to weekly intervals

No Biopsy	*Biopsy*
Continued clinical and laboratory improvement.	Clinical or laboratory relapse after 6 weeks from onset.
	Failure of continued improvement at 10 weeks from onset.
	Failure of complete, progressive resolution any time after 10 weeks.

*Developed and reprinted by permission of J. W. Singleton, M.D., Associate Professor of Medicine, University of Colorado Medical Center.

PLAN:

Patient education
Gamma globulin

Gamma globulin is recommended for contacts of patients with H Bag negative hepatitis. Although this does not prevent development of the disease, it may attenuate the course. There is no contraindication for giving gamma globulin to contacts of HBag positive patients, and early evidence shows some protection for this type also. The usual dose is 0.01 cc./lb. of body weight up to 2 cc.

Prevention of spread

Prevention of spread is identical for both types; the virus is probably present in all body secretions. Therefore, advise the patient to avoid new, personal and intimate contacts (kissing, intercourse) until liver function tests are near normal. Do not share needles, cigarettes, toothbrushes, etc. Use separate dishes, a dishwasher, if available, or disposables. Restaurant dining is discouraged from a public health standpoint. Thorough hand washing after use of the bathroom, good personal hygiene and keeping the bathroom clean, especially around the toilet, are all important counseling points.

Diet

Encourage a well-balanced diet; there are no dietary restrictions. Nausea is often less of a problem in the morning, and the largest meal of the day should be encouraged at that time. Any food which is tolerated is advised. Adequate fluid intake is also important.

Rest

Continued bed rest is not required. Rather, the patient should rest when tired and not push himself to extremes. Continued exertion does not seem to increase the possibility of development of chronic disease, but may prolong convalescence and increase patient discomfort.

Drugs

Hepatic detoxification of drugs and chemicals is impaired in patients with liver disease. Drug effects may therefore be augmented and prolonged, since higher blood levels are maintained for longer periods of time. All drugs used by the patient must be known to the clinician, and hepatotoxicity evaluated. This includes laxatives, antibiotics, alcohol and birth control pills. These and other drugs can cause liver damage and reactivation of symptoms. It is best to avoid chemicals used in the work environment. Besides causing patient distress, these cloud the picture in evaluating chronicity and may prolong the course of illness.

Blood donation

With present knowledge, no person who has had either type of hepatitis should donate blood.

Work disposition

No work for approximately 2 weeks. This depends largely on the amount of physical labor involved, the opportunity to work part time, amount of public contact and subjective symptoms. Food handlers who are HBag positive should not return to work until their HBag has returned to negative.

Return to clinic

Weekly for the first 2 or 3 weeks depending on the patient's course and symptoms. Patients must, if at all possible, be followed until liver function tests return to normal. People over 40 tend to have more difficulty and need closer follow-up. Phone contact with results of lab studies is satisfactory if the patient is feeling well.

BIBLIOGRAPHY

Beeson, Paul B., and Walsh McDermott: *Cecil-Loeb Textbook of Medicine*, 14th ed., Philadelphia: Saunders, 1975.

Wintrobe, M. W. et al. (eds.): *Harrison's Principles of Medicine*, 7th ed., New York: McGraw-Hill, 1974.

NOTES

Chapter 17

Hypertension

HYPERTENSION PROTOCOL

Hypertension without known cause is described as essential hypertension. This refers to a person with systolic readings over 140 mm. Hg and/or diastolic readings greater than 90 mm. Hg on at least three separate occasions.

Subjective information is difficult to evaluate, as the person may be totally asymptomatic, even with extremely elevated pressures, and symptoms the patient does have (e.g. headache) may not be due to the hypertension.

HYPERTENSION WORKSHEET

SUBJECTIVE DATA:

DESCRIBE POSITIVE RESPONSES
(Include Onset, Severity, Duration, Location)

Yes *No*

____ ____ Headaches: _____

____ ____ Dizziness or lightheadedness: _____

____ ____ Shortness of breath: _____

____ ____ Paroxysmal nocturnal dyspnea: _____

____ ____ Cough:

Productive: _____

Sputum (describe): _____

—— —— Edema: _____

—— —— Chest pain:

             Related to: _____

—— —— Drug side effects: _____

—— —— Altered state of well being: _____

—— —— Medications: _____

_____

_____

SUBJECTIVE RATIONALE:

Epistaxis

Do not specifically inquire regarding this, as it is not related to hypertension. Many patients believe a nosebleed means their blood pressure is out of control, and become anxious. Give reassurance or initiate measures for control, if indicated.

Headaches

Poorly correlated with fluctuations in daily blood pressures. May be related to uncontrolled hypertension with diastolic of 120 mm. Hg or greater. Occur in early AM in occipital area and wear off during the day (see Headache Protocol).

Dizziness or lightheadedness

May be due to side effects of medication or postural hypotension. May be associated with nervousness, and is hard to evaluate. Transient changes in intracranial vasculature (e.g. transient ischemic attacks) may cause dizziness. Common in older people with momentary failure of

HYPERTENSION FLOW SHEET

Name
I.D. No.
Age or birthdate

Examination	Dates						
Weight							
BP 5 minutes Reclining							
BP 2 minutes Standing							
Pulse							
Chest Exam							
Cardiac Exam							
Pedal Edema							
Fundi							

Medications	Diet					
Lab and X-Ray Exam Data	Electrolytes					
	Urinalysis					
	CBC					
	Electrocardiogram					
	Chest x-ray exam					
Health Maintenance						
	Pap Smear					
	M.D. Visit					

reflex vasoconstriction in the legs in overcoming the pooling effect of gravity on the circulating blood. Also is a side-effect of some medications. Hypotension caused by over-medication can diminish cerebral blood flow, simulating encephalopathy. Symptoms disappear when drug dosage is lowered and blood pressure rises.

Shortness of breath
Paroxysmal nocturnal dyspnea
Cough
Edema

These are due to left ventricular failure. Dyspnea occurs with transudation of fluid into the interstitial tissues and alveoli of the lungs; high pressure in the pulmonary veins and capillaries is responsible for this phenomenon. Edema is due to secondary right ventricular failure.

Chest pain

Can be anginal, anxietal or musculoskeletal. Angina is related to hypoxia of the myocardium from diminution or cessation of blood flow (see Chest Pain Protocol).

Drug side effects

Each medication and combination of medications has several potential side effects. Many symptoms are drug related, but the clinician must be careful not to suggest symptoms to the patient (see Table 17-1).

Altered state of well being

A nonspecific finding, but may be the only clue that a more detailed evaluation is needed.

Medications

In this section you should record the way the patient is taking his medicine. This may be different than what was ordered and recorded on the flow sheet.

Examination
Weight

All patients should be encouraged to maintain ideal body weight. Decreased weight does not always result in decreased blood pressure, although some patients may be able to discontinue antihypertensives as their weight reaches normal. Sudden increased weight may herald congestive heart failure. Salt overload with impaired renal function causes transudation of fluid into tissue spaces, with resultant edema and weight gain.

BP reclining
5 minutes
BP standing
2 minutes

Use large (leg) cuff on obese or extremely muscular arm. Apprehension, even slight, can raise blood pressure; resting the patient can help him relax. Position of patient for blood pressure check should be consistent for long term follow-up. Several drugs, notably guanethidine (Ismelin), can cause symptomatic postural hypotension. This drug causes reduced cardiac output in its early use and reduced peripheral resistance with continued therapy. Methyldopa may cause orthostatic hypotension, but this usually disappears with continued therapy. Hypovolemia can cause a drop in standing blood pressure and may be due to drugs which cause water or electrolyte depletion.

Pulse

A normal sinus rhythm is desired. Arrhythmias related to hypertension or drug treatment, or both, can be recognized and counted. Premature ventricular contractions (PVC's) up to 5 a minute are usually

TABLE 17-1
DRUGS USED IN TREATMENT OF HYPERTENSION—LISTED ACCORDING TO SITE OF ACTION

Site of action	Drug	Dosage	Indications	Contraindications	Frequent or peculiar side effects
Central	Clonidine	Oral: 0.2–0.6 mg q.i.d.	Mild to moderate hypertension, renal disease with hypertension		Postural hypotension, drowsiness, dry mouth
	Alpha-methyldopa (also acts by blocking sympathetic nerves)	Oral: 250–750 mg t.i.d.–q.i.d. IV: 500–1000 mg q.4–6 h. (tolerance may develop)	Mild to moderate hypertension (oral), malignant hypertension (IV), in patients who cannot take oral treatment, renal disease with hypertension	Pheochromocytoma, active hepatic disease, during MAO inhibitor administration	Postural hypotension, sedation, fatigue, diarrhea, impaired ejaculation, fever, gynecomastia, lactation, positive Coombs tests (Occasionally associated with hemolysis)
	Sedatives and tranquilizers Phenobarbital	Oral: 15–30 mg t.i.d.–q.i.d.	Tense or anxious patient with hypertension		Drowsiness, fatigue
	Diazepam	Oral: 2–10 mg q.i.d.			
Ganglions	Trimethaphan Pentolinium	IV: 1–10 mg/min IV: 1–5 mg/min IM: 2–5 mg q.2–6 h.	Severe or malignant hypertension	Severe coronary artery disease, cerebrovascular insufficiency, diabetes mellitus (on hypoglycemic therapy), glaucoma, prostatism	Postural hypotension, visual symptoms, dry mouth, constipation, urinary retention, impotence
	Mecamylamine	Oral: 2.5–10 mg q.8–12 h. (most completely absorbed of oral blocking agents)			Tremors, confusion
Nerve endings	Rauwolfia alkaloids		Mild to moderate hypertension in young patients	Pheochromocytoma, peptic ulcer, depression, during MAO inhibitor administration	Depression, nightmares, nasal congestion, dyspepsia, diarrhea, impotence

	Drug	Dosage	Use	Contraindications	Side Effects
	Reserpine	Oral: 0.1–0.5 mg q.d.			
	Guanethidine	Oral: 10–300 mg q.d.	Severe hypertension	Pheochromocytoma, severe coronary artery disease, cerebrovascular insufficiency, during MAO inhibitor administration	Postural hypotension, bradycardia, dry mouth, diarrhea, impaired ejaculation, fluid retention
	Pargyline	Oral: 10–100 mg q.d.	Depressed patient with moderate to severe hypertension	Pheochromocytoma, severe coronary artery disease, cerebrovascular insufficiency, hyperthyroidism, paranoid schizophrenia, during administration of other drugs that act at same site	Postural hypotension, insomnia, nightmares, diarrhea, muscle twitching, acute hypertension (induced by tyramine-containing foods and certain drugs)
Alpha receptors	Phentolamine	IV: 1–5 mg	Suspected or proved pheochromocytoma		Tachycardia, weakness, dizziness, flushing
	Phenoxybenzamine	Oral: 10–50 mg q.d.–b.i.d., (tolerance may develop)	Proved pheochromocytoma	Severe coronary artery disease	Postural hypotension, tachycardia, miosis, nasal congestion, dry mouth
Beta receptors	Propranolol	Oral: 10–40 mg q.i.d.	Mild hypertension (especially with evidence for hyperdynamic circulation), adjunct to hydralazine therapy, pheochromocytoma	Congestive heart failure, asthma, diabetes mellitus (on hypoglycemic therapy), during MAO inhibitor administration	Dizziness, depression bronchospasm, nausea, vomiting, diarrhea, constipation, heart failure
Vascular smooth muscle	Hydralazine	Oral: 10–50 mg q.i.d. IV or IM: 10–50 mg q.6 h. (tolerance may develop)	As adjunct in treatment of moderate to severe hypertension (oral), malignant hypertension (IV or IM), renal disease with hypertension	Lupus erythematosus, severe coronary artery disease, mitral valvular rheumatic heart	Headache, tachycardia, angina pectoris, anorexia, nausea, vomiting, diarrhea, lupus syndrome

TABLE 17-1 (Continued)

DRUGS USED IN TREATMENT OF HYPERTENSION—LISTED ACCORDING TO SITE OF ACTION

Site of action	Drug	Dosage	Indications	Contraindications	Frequent or peculiar side effects
	Diazoxide	IV: 300 mg rapidly	Severe or malignant hypertension	Diabetes mellitus, hyperuricemia, congestive heart failure	Hyperglycemia, hyperuricemia, sodium retention
	Rauwolfia alkaloids Reserpine	IM: 2.5–5 mg q. 6 h.	Malignant hypertension	Pheochromocytoma, during MAO inhibitor administration	Lethargy, nasal congestion, facial flushing, extrapyramidal signs
Renal tubule	Thiazides		Mild hypertension, as adjunct in treatment of moderate to severe hypertension	Diabetes mellitus, hyperuricemia, primary aldosteronism	Potassium depletion, hyperglycemia, hyperuricemia, dermatitis, purpura
	Hydrochlorothiazide	Oral: 25–50 mg q.d.–b.i.d.			
	Furosemide	Oral: 20–40 mg q.d.–b.i.d.	Mild hypertension	Hyperuricemia, primary aldosteronism	Potassium depletion, hyperuricemia, nausea, vomiting, diarrhea
	Ethacrynic acid	Oral: 25–50 mg q.d.–b.i.d.	Mild hypertension	Hyperuricemia, primary aldosteronism	Potassium depletion, hyperuricemia, diarrhea
	Spironolactone	Oral: 25–100 mg t.i.d.–q.i.d.	Hypertension due to hypermineralocorticoidism, adjunct to thiazide therapy	Renal failure	Hyperuricemia, diarrhea, gynecomastia, menstrual irregularities
	Triamterine	Oral: 100 mg q.d.–t.i.d.	Hypertension due to hypermineralocorticoidism, adjunct to thiazide therapy	Renal failure	Hyperkalemia, nausea, vomiting, leg cramps

From Wintrobe's *Harrison's Principles of Internal Medicine*, 7th ed. © 1974, McGraw-Hill Book Co. Used with permission of McGraw-Hill Book Co.

acceptable. This can be normal to that individual or caused by such things as caffeine. Increased PVC's or tachycardia can mean electrolyte imbalance or side-effects of medications which alter cardiac activity. Cardiac rate is also related to unconscious nervous control.

Chest exam

Listen for rales or rhonchi which may herald congestive heart failure. These occur as a result of capillary congestion causing transudation of fluid into the air spaces and interstitial tissues of the lungs.

Cardiac exam

A shift of the point of maximal impulse to the left usually indicates left ventricular enlargement (LVH), which is common in hypertensives. LVH occurs as a result of the added workload of the heart in pumping against increased peripheral resistance. The ventricle also dilates because it fails to empty normally in systole. The appearance of an arrhythmia or new murmur calls for physician consultation. Arrhythmias can be due to electrolyte imbalance or side effects of medications.

Pedal edema

Presence of edema, pitting or non-pitting, indicates cardiac failure and salt overload. Weight may increase as much as 10 % before pitting edema occurs. Poor emptying of the heart during systole promotes an accumulation of blood in the heart and venous circulation. Edema accumulates in the legs largely because of posture and the effect of gravity.

Fundi

Look for arterio-venous (A-V) nicking, exudates or hemorrhages which occur with uncontrolled hypertension. Funduscopic changes are the earliest indication of end-organ disease. Record what is seen or draw a diagram. Look for diminution in the caliber of small vessels most distal from the disc. Segmental constriction of the arterioles is a permanent lesion and is characteristic of significant diastolic hypertension. Tortuosity of large vessels close to the disc is of little importance. To be significant, A-V nicking must occur at least 1 disc diameter from the edge of the optic disc. This is a permanent change. Increased light reflex signifies thickening of the vessel walls. Small, flame-like hemorrhages and white exudates are advanced changes but may be reversible. Papilledema is a serious prognostic sign of advanced disease and demands immediate hospitalization and treatment.

Medication

A regular tabulation of the patient's medication is a must. When recorded on a flow sheet, changes in medication and their effects in blood pressure can be easily observed.

Diet

Should be salt-restricted, that is, no added salt. 500 mg. to 1 gm. sodium diet is the ideal, but requires a great deal of patient compliance and less than 2 gm. is usually not practical. Caloric intake should be adjusted for weight maintenance or reduction as indicated. Obese patients have an added risk for coronary artery disease. Elevated lipids are an added risk. Fasting cholesterol and triglycerides need monitoring and appropriate adjustment of diet should be made accordingly.

Lab and X-Ray Exam Data

Electrolytes
Blood sugar
Uric acid

Those which will be monitored depend on medications used. Electrolytes, especially potassium, need to be checked when using most diuretics. Draw these at the start of therapy, every 6-8 weeks until stable, and at least every 6 months thereafter. Antihypertensive drugs may also cause elevated blood sugar and uric acid which should be checked as above.

Urinalysis

Renal parenchymal disease may be the underlying cause of hypertension which is being controlled by medications. Arterial nephrosclerosis may precede or follow hypertension. Look for renal involvement by the appearance of casts or proteinuria.

CBC

Perform frequently with some medications, notably Methyldopa, which may cause acquired hemolytic anemia. Interval should otherwise be determined by agreement with physician, and may depend on other underlying diseases the patient has.

EKG

Indicated if chest symptoms or auscultatory changes occur. Allows documentation of cardiac status which should correlate with objective findings. Do at least yearly.

Chest x-ray exam | Indicated if chest symptoms or auscultatory changes occurs. Aids in documentation of objective physical findings, e.g. fluid. Useful in monitoring cardiac size and vascular changes. Do at least yearly.

Health Maintenance
Pap smear | Perform yearly.

M.D. visit | Frequency must be established by N.P./M.D. team, and a mutually agreed upon protocol established. Consultation should be sought with blood pressures greater than 160/110 despite consistent medication ingestion, change of medication or dosage, new objective or subjective findings.

ASSESSMENT: | The goal is control of blood pressure with the least amount of medicine. Patients must be aware that other medications can cause or aggravate hypertension, notably over the counter sympathomimetics and birth control pills. Patients should not only know the names of their medications but should carry a card listing them in case of an emergency.

Medication change | Requires physician consultation. See Table I for list of commonly used medicines.

PLAN:
Interval of visit | This depends on degree of blood pressure control and reliability of the patient. During initiation of therapy and drug change, the patient should be seen every 2-3

weeks. Patients who are reliable in taking their drugs, and who are in good control on established regimens, may be followed every 6 months.

To commit a person to a lifetime of medications and expect compliance requires ingenuity and compassion. The nurse practitioner, through concern and consistent care, can help reduce the morbidity and mortality from uncontrolled hypertension.

BIBLIOGRAPHY

Beeson, Paul B., and Walsh McDermott: *Cecil-Loeb Textbook of Medicine,* 14th ed., Philadelphia: Saunders, 1975.

Wintrobe, M. W., et al. (eds.): *Harrison's Principles of Internal Medicine,* 7th ed., New York: McGraw-Hill, 1974.

Chapter 18

Rheumatoid arthritis

RHEUMATOID ARTHRITIS PROTOCOL

Rheumatoid arthritis is a systemic disease characterized by inflammation of the synovial membrane of diarthrodial joints, and is frequently accompanied by a variety of extra-articular manifestations. The synovial inflammation eventually results in the destruction of joint cartilage and supporting structures. In caring for the patient with rheumatoid arthritis, it is important to remember that the natural course of the disease is characterized by periods of spontaneous remissions and exacerbations.

The parameters monitored in this protocol relate to the general management of the disease and include the use of gold therapy.

Management goals for the patient with rheumatoid arthritis include:

1. Decrease pain and inflammation
2. Maintain function
3. Prevent deformity
4. Increase understanding of the disease and rationale for the management regime

RHEUMATOID ARTHRITIS WORKSHEET

SUBJECTIVE DATA:

DESCRIBE POSITIVE RESPONSES
(Include Onset, Severity, Duration, Location)

ARTHRITIS STATUS:

Yes   No

____ ____ Heat, redness, swelling of joints: _____

___ ___ Loss of function: _____

___ ___ Increased pain:_____

___ ___ Increased AM stiffness:

                Duration: _____

                Relieved by: _____

GENERAL:
Yes   No

                           Name   How taking

___ ___ Medications _____   _____

                                 _____   _____

                                 _____   _____

                                 _____   _____

___ ___ Drug side effects: _____

PATIENT ON GOLD THERAPY

MEDIA TOXICITY:
Yes   No

___ ___ Urticaria: _____

___ ___ Flushing: _____

___ ___ Weakness: _____

___ ___ Palpitations: _____

GOLD TOXICITY:
Yes   No

___ ___ Rash/pruritus: _____

___ ___ Mouth/throat ulcers: _____

RHEUMATOID ARTHRITIS FLOW SHEET

Name
I.D. No.
Age

Examination							
Dates							
Blood Pressure							
Weight							
Joint Exam/ Inflammatory Index							
M.D. Visit							
Gold Preparation							

Medications	(Total Dose)					
Lab Data	WBC					
	Hct/HGB					
	Urine Protein					
	Joint X-rays					
Health Maintenance						
	Pap Smear					
	Chest X-ray exam					

_____ _____ Recent diarrhea: _____

_____ _____ Vision changes: _____

_____ _____ Increasing bruising: _____

_____ _____ Sudden change in arthritis status: _____

SUBJECTIVE RATIONALE:

Heat, redness, swelling of joints	Indicators of inflammation. History of these signs and symptoms is a good indication of the amount of synovitis the patient is experiencing.
Loss of function	Inability to perform certain previously carried out tasks or activities of daily living provides information regarding progression of disease.
Increased pain Increased AM stiffness	Degree of pain and morning stiffness usually correlate with degree of synovial inflammation.
General Medications	This information is useful in determining patient compliance, identifying questions related to drug side effects or benefits, determining the frequency and type of drug use (such as pain medications) and evaluating other symptoms in the context of this information.
Drug side effects	Care giver should ask specific questions based on medications patient is taking, to determine if adverse reactions warrant discontinuance of drug.
Patient on Gold Therapy	Gold therapy is usually initiated when the disease continues to pro-

2nd and 3rd week respectively. If tolerated, then 50 mgm. is given (IM) weekly until a good response is reached. This usually does not occur until 400-600 mgm. total dose is achieved. Injections may then be stretched out to every 2 weeks for 3-4 times, and then every 3 to 4 weeks according to the response of the patient. Once a beneficial response to gold is achieved (2/3 will have some benefit) the patient receives maintenance injections (50 mgm.) on a monthly basis.

Laboratory/X-Ray Exam Data
CBC and differential monthly
WBC ⎱
Hct ⎰ before each
Hgb ⎰ gold injection

Anemia is frequently present, due to mild bone marrow suppression accompanying chronic illness; this may be compounded by chronic gastrointestinal blood loss from ulcerogenic medications such as acetylsalicylic acid and indomethacin. Eosinophilia may precede impending gold toxicity.

Urine protein

With nephrotoxicity due to gold, the glomerular membrane becomes more permeable, and plasma proteins are allowed to pass through. This is manifested as proteinuria. Microscopic hematuria may also be seen. This toxicity may progress to nephrotic syndrome if gold is not stopped. However, with temporary discontinuation of the drug, the proteinuria and hematuria are usually reversible, and gold may be resumed with caution.

Joint x-ray exams

May be ordered on specific joints on a yearly basis to monitor course of disease radiographically. Hand films are often used for this purpose.

Health Maintenance

See Health Maintenance Chapter.

Pap smear
Chest x-ray exam
Health hazard data

If the patient is receiving primary care in your setting, guidelines should be established for obtaining health maintenance data.

ASSESSMENT:

Goals of management include decreasing pain and inflammation, maintaining function and preventing deformity.

Toxic manifestations to gold, such as rash, itching, aphthous ulcers usually abate with temporary discontinuance of the drug. Gold may be restarted at lower or the same dosages upon disappearance of the toxic signs.

Some of the other drugs frequently used in the management of rheumatoid arthritis, and their common side-effects, are listed below:

Drugs	*Side Effects*
Acetylsalicylic acid (aspirin)	Gastric irritation, tinnitus. Potentiates anticoagulant effect.
Antimalarials (Plaquenil/ Hydroxy-chloroquine)	Retinal vasculitis. Condition may progress even after discontinuance of drug. Frequent ophthalmologic examinations are mandatory for patients on these drugs.
Indomethacin (Indocin)	Gastrointestinal irritation, nausea and vomiting, epigastric pain, peptic ulcer, headache, vertigo, dizziness. Rarely, a mild pruritic macular dermatitis may occur.

Drugs	Side Effects
Ibuprofen (Motrin)	Mainly gastrointestinal irritation, although less frequent than with other anti-inflammatories. Pruritus, maculopapular and vesiculobullous eruptions; dizziness; rarely amblyopia.
Phenylbutazone (Butazolidin)	Sodium retention, rash, peptic ulcer, bone marrow suppression. Potentiates anticoagulant effect. Macular dermatitis is rare.

While evaluating response to treatment, it is important to remember that emotional adjustment to the disease must also be continuously assessed and managed.

PLAN:

Patient education

Understanding the disease and the plan of therapy is essential if the patient is to comply with treatment over many years. Patients should know their medications by name, the benefits to expect from each and the side effects which may occur. Special instructions, such as taking acetylsalicylic acid and anti-inflammatories with food, and observing stool color for melena, should be periodically reinforced.

BIBLIOGRAPHY

Ehrlich, George E.: *Total Management of the Arthritic Patient,* Philadelphia: Lippincott, 1973.

Hollander, Joseph Lee: *Arthritis and Allied Conditions,* Philadelphia: Lea and Febiger, 8th ed., 1972.

Mason, Michael, and H. L. F. Currey: *Clinical Rheumatology,* Philadelphia: Lippincott, 1970.

Primer on the Rheumatic Diseases, 7th ed., 1973. The Arthritis Foundation.

NOTES

NOTES

Health
maintenance

Chapter 19

Health maintenance
and health
hazard appraisal

The area of health care relating to prevention of disease and illness and to health maintenance is often neglected, even though it is a very important aspect of care. Unfortunately, few people are motivated to seek health maintenance care in the absence of illness. Thus, when a person does come to a health care setting for a specific problem, the time should be utilized to make an assessment of his health status as a whole. It provides an opportunity to identify precursors of illness that can be modified, possibly preventing future illness. Positive factors that contribute to health can also be identified and reinforced.

The other chapters covered the subjective and objective information needed to identify and correctly assess specific common problems and the treatment and patient education appropriate for these problems. The approach used with the patient during health care teaching is probably the most important factor influencing compliance and thus follow-through and successful treatment. To individualize patient care and teaching, one needs to constantly utilize a knowledge of behavioral sciences. Information needed for the data base in general involves identification of:

1. the person's concept of health and illness;
2. his motivation for seeking health care;
3. the priorities in his life relating to himself and his family;
4. life-style patterns which point to strengths that contribute to his health;
5. life-style patterns that are risk factors for specific disease/accident occurrences, and;
6. an assessment of his ability to understand what is taught.

These are important pieces of information for the data base, not only to provide the necessary care for specific acute or chronic health problems, but also to provide health maintenance care.

What is health or wellness? This is a complex question, and the answer cannot be provided here. Each person will have a different definition of what health or wellness is; it does not necessarily mean just the absence of disease. It is the individual's concept of health and illness that forms the basis for his motivation toward health care. Many people seek health care only when they are in some way incapacitated by illness or disease. However, a small number seek help when no disease is present. Although no physical problem can be identified, they perceive that a problem exists. This group is often defined as the "worried well."

Motivation in seeking health care is directly related to life priorities, and economics often plays a vital role. A person who perceives himself as healthy may not see preventive care as a priority because of other needs in his life. This individual may only seek health care when illness interferes with these priorities.

The individual's concept of the health care provider's role is another important motivating factor. He may perceive the "role" only as illness-oriented and not as providing health or preventive care. Thus, when the person does seek help, for whatever reason, the health care provider must try to provide complete care, including both treatment of illness and maintenance of health.

A priority of health care does need to be treatment of illness when it is present. As long as the person is ill, his priority will be to get well. Prevention of subsequent illness will probably not be his priority at this time. However, the health care provider can look to the future and begin a health status assessment and plan. It is an appropriate time to let the patient know his strengths and those positive aspects of his life-style that will contribute to future health. It is a time to let the patient know that health care does include prevention. And, for the person who is one of the "worried well," providing information about his health status as a whole, his strengths and risks, will not only reassure him, but also give him a goal to reach to reduce risks for possible future disease.

Areas to assess in the person's life style include, but are not limited to:

1. ability to cope with everyday stresses at work and at home. What is his pattern of coping or adapting to changes in his life? Does he experience extreme mood swings? Is he often depressed?

2. dietary habits. Does he eat regular, well-balanced meals? Does he take time to eat slowly in a relaxed atmosphere? Does he over- or under-eat? Is he under- or overweight? Does he consume many caffeine-containing beverages? Does his diet include large amounts of high-cholesterol and triglyceride foods?

3. level of activity. Does he spend time exercising, either in his work or in recreational activities?

4. driving habits. When he drives, does he use a seat belt? Does he drive within the speed limit?

5. alcohol consumption. What are his drinking habits? Does he drive when drinking?

6. use of tobacco. Does he use tobacco in any form? Specifically, does he smoke cigarettes? If so, how many per day?

Many of these habits have been found to be precursors of diseases which are leading causes of death in certain age, sex and race categories.[1] Precursors are forerunners of disease; they are risks which directly contribute to the development of disease, and thus, may be directly or indirectly related to death. A person's life-style may be increasing his risk for specific disease entities. If he can understand that changing these habits can reduce his risk for a specific disease, he may be motivated to modify his life-style.

We need to be aware of these risk factors in each person we see for health care. If we know the leading cause of death for the average person of the same age, sex and race, we can be particularly alert to risk factors in a given individual. And, conversely, if the risk factors are not present, we can reinforce habits which positively contribute to that individual's health.

The following information gives some examples of behavior or conditions related to leading causes of death. The average risk for each of the causes of death varies for people of different age, sex and race groups. Also illustrated is the degree to which the risk factor can be decreased after successful health teaching, and modification of life-style habits. The list is not exhaustive, but will demonstrate a few areas where health care teaching and intervention by the nurse practitioner can be used in preventive care.

[1]Robbins, Lewis G., and Jack H. Hall: *How to Practice Prospective Medicine,* Indianapolis, Indiana: Methodist Hospital of Indiana, 1970.

Cause of Death	Precursor	Risk Factor	Reduction of Risk Possible with Intervention
Suicide	If person is often *depressed*, he is at risk for suicide as cause of death.	In relation to the average person, he is at 2½ times greater risk for suicide	With counseling that results in fewer episodes and less severe depression, his risk for suicide can be decreased to that of the average person.
ASHD	A person who is *overweight* is at greater risk for death from arteriosclerotic heart disease.	If he is 75% overweight, his risk is 2½ times greater than the average person. At 50 % overweight, his risk is 1½ times that of the average person.	A person at average weight, or up to 15 % overweight, is at average risk for death from arteriosclerotic heart disease. Thus, the person who is overweight can decrease his risk by weight reduction.
ASHD	A person who is *sedentary* at work and leisure is at greater risk for death due to arteriosclerotic heart disease.	His risk is nearly 1½ times that of the average person.	Walking ½ to 1½ miles per day, or comparable activity, can reduce his risk to average. Increasing activity even more can reduce *his* risk to *below* that of the average person.
ASHD	A person who smokes *cigarettes* is at risk for death due to arteriosclerotic heart disease.	If he smokes a pack or more per day he may be 1½–2 times the average risk.	Reducing smoking to below ½ pack per day can reduce the risk somewhat. If he has stopped smoking for 10 years (or has never smoked) his risk is below average.

Vehicle accidents	If *seat belts* are used less than 10 % of the time, the person is at greater risk for death by vehicle accidents.	This person's risk is 1.1 times the average risk.	Use of seat belts 75-100 % of the time can reduce the risk to below that of the average person.
Vehicle accidents	A person who drinks *alcohol* is at greater risk for death by motor vehicle accidents, either while driving or as a pedestrian.		A nondrinker has only ½ times the risk of the average person who drinks 3-6 drinks per week. Thus, if the person does not drink either while driving or when a pedestrian, his risk for death by motor vehicle accidents can be reduced to below average.
	Heavy drinking: 25-40 drinks per week.	Risk is 5 times greater than the average person's risk.	
	Social drinking: 7-24 drinks per week.	Risk is twice that of the average person.	
Cirrhosis	A person who drinks *alcohol* is at greater risk for death due to cirrhosis. His risk increases with an increase in drinking.		

Cause of Death	Precursor	Risk Factor	Reduction of Risk Possible with Intervention
Cirrhosis	"Social drinker": more than 7 drinks per week.	This person's risk for cirrhosis is greater than the average person who drinks 3-6 drinks per week.	A person who drinks 3-6 drinks per week is at average risk. If he drinks less than 3 drinks, he is at lower than average risk.
	"Heavy drinker": over 24 drinks per week.	His risk can be as high as 5 times that of the average person.	
CNS vascular lesions	A person who smokes *cigarettes*, no matter how many, is at greater risk for death due to vascular lesions affecting the central nervous system	His risk is 1½ times that of the average person.	If he stops smoking he can reduce his risk to average. Those who have never smoked are at below average risk.
Lung cancer	A person who smokes 1-2 packs of *cigarettes* per day is at greater risk for death due to cancer of the lung.	His risk is 1½ to 2 times that of the average person.	A person who stops smoking can eventually reduce his risk for cancer of the lung; the risk factor decreases each year he has stopped. The nonsmoker is at very low risk for lung cancer.

The nurse practitioner can use the above information in teaching how modification of life-style patterns can reduce risk for death from a specific disease. For instance, Mr. X is a 40 year old white male who is 25% overweight, has a sedentary job and very little recreational activity. He likes to golf but usually rides a cart instead of walking the course. He also smokes about one pack of cigarettes a day. Assuming all other risk factors are average, Mr. X has over 3 times the risk of the average man his age for death due to arteriosclerotic heart disease. If this man would stop smoking, lose weight so he is no more than 15 % overweight and begin to walk ½ to 1½ miles per day or take comparable exercise, he could reduce his risk for death from arteriosclerotic heart disease to approximately average. In fact, his risk would be slightly under the average risk.

The life style pattern of a person may also affect his health status, although not directly cause death. For example, what a person eats can not only affect his weight but also cause other health problems, such as gastric disturbances from caffeine containing drinks. Daily dental hygiene habits can affect health, as periodontal diseases are quite prevalent.

Health care providers cannot change a person's life-style. However, by presenting information about risks for illness and disease in an individualized way, health care teaching may have increased meaning for a person, and could be the motivating factor for modifying life-style and thus reducing risks. By utilizing knowledge of the behavioral sciences, as well as scientific data, health care providers can facilitate learning for the patient and help *him* maintain *his* health.

BIBLIOGRAPHY

Bruhn, John G.: "The Diagnosis of Normality," *Texas Reports on Biology and Medicine,* vol. 32, pp. 242-248, Spring 1974.

Bruhn, John G.: "The Maintenance of Wellness," *Continuing Education,* pp. 52-56, January 1975.

Garfield, Sidney R.: "The Delivery of Medical Care," *Scientific American,* vol. 222, pp. 15-23, April 1970.

Robbins, Lewis C., and Jack H. Hall: *How to Practice Prospective Medicine,* Indianapolis, Indiana: Methodist Hospital of Indiana, 1970.

Index